EKGs for the Nurse Practitioner and Physician Assistant

Maureen A. Knechtel, MPAS, PA-C, received a bachelor's degree in health sciences and a master's degree in physician assistant studies from Duquesne University in Pittsburgh, Pennsylvania. Upon completion of her training in 2005, she began her career as a cardiology physician assistant with Pittsburgh Cardiac and Vascular Associates. Since 2008, she has been fortunate to pursue her dream as an electrophysiology physician assistant with The Wellmont Cardiovascular Associates Heart Institute in Kingsport, Tennessee. She teaches EKG recognition and interpretation to both physician assistants and nurse practitioners and has been a guest lecturer nationally and locally on topics including chronic angina, ischemic heart disease in women, hypertension, and mixed hyperlipidemia. She serves as a primary preceptor for several local physician assistant and nurse practitioner programs. Maureen is a fellow member of the American Academy of Physician Assistants and the Tennessee Academy of Physician Assistants.

EKGs for the Nurse Practitioner and Physician Assistant

MAUREEN A. KNECHTEL, MPAS, PA-C

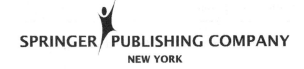

SPRINGER PUBLISHING COMPANY
NEW YORK

Springer Publishing Company, LLC
11 West 42nd Street
New York, NY 10036
www.springerpub.com

Acquisitions Editor: Margaret Zuccarini
Composition: diacriTech

ISBN: 9780826199560
Ebook ISBN: 9780826199577

16/5

The author and the publisher of this Work have made every effort to use sources believed to be reliable to provide information that is accurate and compatible with the standards generally accepted at the time of publication. Because medical science is continually advancing, our knowledge base continues to expand. Therefore, as new information becomes available, changes in procedures become necessary. We recommend that the reader always consult current research and specific institutional policies before performing any clinical procedure. The author and publisher shall not be liable for any special, consequential, or exemplary damages resulting, in whole or in part, from the readers' use of, or reliance on, the information contained in this book. The publisher has no responsibility for the persistence or accuracy of URLs for external or third-party Internet websites referred to in this publication and does not guarantee that any content on such websites is, or will remain, accurate or appropriate.

Library of Congress Cataloging-in-Publication Data

Knechtel, Maureen A.
  EKG interpretation for the physician assistant and nurse practitioner / Maureen A. Knechtel.
      p. ; cm.
  ISBN 978-0-8261-9956-0—ISBN 978-0-8261-9957-7 (e-book)
  I. Title.
  [DNLM: 1. Electrocardiography—methods. 2. Electrocardiography—nursing.
3. Heart Diseases—diagnosis. 4. Heart Diseases—nursing. WG 140]
  RC683.5.E5
  616.1'207547—dc23
                              2013000907

Special discounts on bulk quantities of our books are available to corporations, professional associations, pharmaceutical companies, health care organizations, and other qualifying groups. If you are interested in a custom book, including chapters from more than one of our titles, we can provide that service as well.
For details, please contact:
Special Sales Department, Springer Publishing Company, LLC
11 West 42nd Street, 15th Floor, New York, NY 10036-8002
Phone: 877-687-7476 or 212-431-4370; Fax: 212-941-7842
E-mail: sales@springerpub.com

Printed in the United States of America by Bradford and Bigelow.

To Dr. Arun Rao, Dr. Gregory Jones, and Dr. James Merrill: Thank you for your patience and wisdom in teaching me everything I know about EKGs.

To Jim and Kathy Moran: Thank you for a lifetime of encouragement and motivation.

To Dave: The better half of Team Knechtel—Thank you for your constant love and support.

Contents

Preface

This book is written for the nurse practitioner and physician assistant, but it is intended for any health care provider who is attempting to master the EKG. EKGs are frequently seen as daunting to conquer, and we are often content to simply learn the basics and move on with the rest of our training. In my opinion, the problem lies in the way EKGs are presented. The facts are laid out in books filled with numbers and lines, and we find ourselves memorizing the material, perhaps in hopes of simply passing a test. The goal of my book is to present not only the facts but also the physiology behind the process. We will review clinical scenarios in which you may see certain abnormalities to allow for a real-life approach. This should lead to less memorizing and more understanding and allow for those facts to transition to everyday clinical use.

With more and more nurse practitioners and physician assistants providing primary care, it is vital to be able to recognize abnormalities early and make appropriate clinical decisions. This book will encompass all major areas of EKG interpretation and prepare you to be confident in your interpretation skills. In taking on the responsibility of providing care for our patients, it is vital to be a master of the EKG no matter what your specialty.

It is imperative to always follow a pattern when interpreting EKGs. You should get into the habit of following the same steps each time so you will be sure not to leave anything out. This will also prevent you from becoming overwhelmed. When you pick up an EKG, you need to be able to quickly pick out the main points: rate, rhythm, axis, block, and infarction. Ask yourself: What is the heart rate? Is the rhythm regular or irregular? Is there heart block? Is there evidence of ischemia or infarction? Note the axis: Is it left, right, or indeterminate? It doesn't matter in what order you review these points. Just find a system that works for you and don't leave anything out. Let's get started.

Maureen A. Knechtel, MPAS, PA-C

1

Introduction to the EKG, Cardiac Anatomy, and Electrical Conduction System

INTRODUCTION

The electrocardiogram (EKG) records the electrical activity of the heart through specialized terminals called electrodes that are placed at distinct locations on the human body surface. Currents are transmitted and recorded based on the location of these electrodes and the relationships that are created between them. The EKG depicts the direction of energy flow through the heart. This electrical cascade begins with stimulation of the individual myocytes and continues on through specialized areas of conducting cells that create the sinus node, atrioventricular (AV) node, bundle of His (pronounced *hiss*), and the bundle branches. Sometimes detours are taken around conduction blocks or scar tissue that may change the appearance of the typical EKG. On completion of this text, you should feel confident in the ability to navigate and interpret this complex road map of electrical activity and move one step closer to becoming a master of the 12-lead EKG.

DEPOLARIZATION AND REPOLARIZATION

The terms **depolarization** and **repolarization** refer to a change in the electrical charge of myocytes involved in conduction. All cardiac cells have a negative resting internal charge. To initiate contraction, a positive charge spreads from the sinus node down through the myocardium. The myocardial cells gain a positive charge, causing them to contract. This process is referred to as depolarization. The cells become repolarized after electrical conduction ends and they regain a negative resting charge (Figure 1.1).

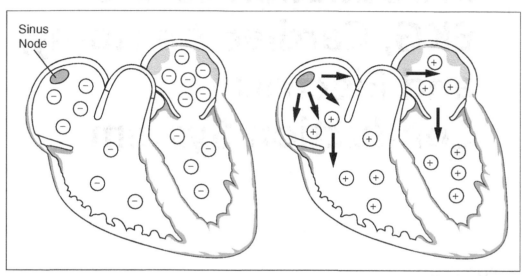

FIGURE 1.1

This electrical activity through the heart is represented on EKG by a P wave, QRS complex, and T wave and the intervals that are created between them. The P wave represents atrial depolarization, the QRS complex represents ventricular depolarization, and the ST segment and T wave together represent the entirety of ventricular repolarization (EKG 1.1).

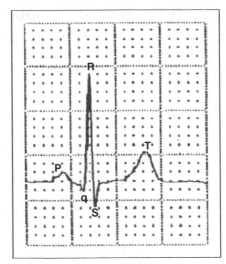

EKG 1.1

EKG complexes appear upright (positive) or downright (negative) based on the flow of electricity toward or away from that area. If electricity spreads toward an area, the EKG complex representing that portion of the myocardium will have an upright appearance because those cells are becoming positive (EKG 1.2). Likewise, if electricity spreads away from an area, the affected EKG complex will have a downward appearance (EKG 1.3).

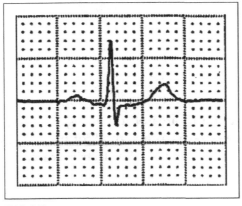

EKG 1.2

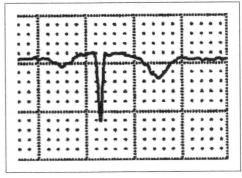

EKG 1.3

The ability of cells to initiate a pacemaker impulse is termed **automaticity**. Areas of cells that generate a pacemaker impulse are termed automaticity foci. Automaticity foci are located in the sinus node, the AV node, and the ventricles. The anatomy of the conduction system is presented below and illustrated in Figure 1.2.

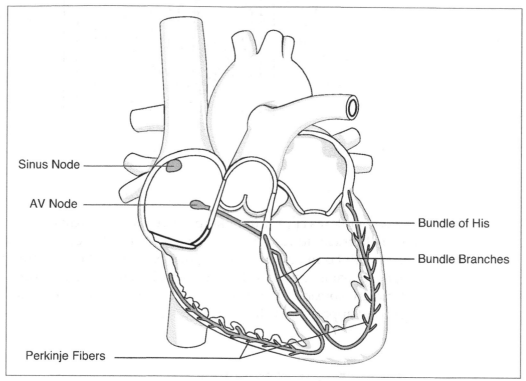

FIGURE 1.2

SINUS NODE

Located in the high right atrium, this area of impulse-generating tissue sits near the entrance of the superior vena cava. Although all of the cells in the atria have the ability to generate an impulse and initiate the electrical cascade, the **sinus node** (also known as sinoatrial [SA] node) sets the pace because it conducts slightly faster than its competitors located more distal in the conduction system. Normal sinus node activity occurs at 60 to 100 beats per minute and is seen on EKG as a P wave. A normal P wave should be monophasic or entirely positive or negative.

Normal sinus activity is reflected on EKG by a positive P wave. A focus originating lower in the atrium can cause inverted P waves. This is referred to as a low atrial focus, and indicates that the normal sinus node has failed to initiate a timely electrical impulse (EKG 1.4).

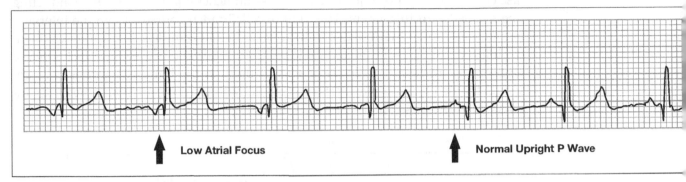

Low Atrial Focus   Normal Upright P Wave

EKG 1.4

ATRIOVENTRICULAR NODE

After the electrical impulse initiates in the right atrium, conduction ripples slowly through both atria toward the **AV node**. It is a compact area of tissue that lies in the interatrial septum near the coronary sinus. This is the electrical connection between the atria and the ventricles and can be thought of as the gatekeeper of electrical impulses that pass through the heart. Conduction must slow here to allow the tricuspid valve and mitral valve to open and the ventricles to fill with blood prior to systole. Activity through the AV node is reflected on EKG as the PR interval.

If the sinus node fails to generate an impulse and initiate the electrical cascade, the AV node has this ability although it will do so at a slower rate. The normal intrinsic firing rate of the AV node without stimulation from elsewhere, that is, the sinus node, is 40 to 60 beats per minute. This rate is telling of a junctional rhythm if it occurs in the absence of P waves.

BUNDLE OF HIS

This area of conducting tissue is just distal to the AV node. Its main purpose is to connect electrical signals from the AV node to the ventricular bundle branches. Electrical activity from the **bundle of His** is not directly reflected on EKG by any specific interval. It is an important anatomical marker in terms of defining the location of a block, specifically second-degree type I versus second-degree type II. Savvy clinicians can impress their colleagues by describing a block as "infra-hisian" in origin. See Chapter 7 for more on this topic.

BUNDLE BRANCHES

The bundle branches are divided into the **right bundle branch and left bundle branch** (Figure 1.3). The left bundle branch is further divided into the left anterior fascicle and the left posterior fascicle. These branches comprise rapidly conducting fibers called **Purkinje fibers**. The right bundle branch courses down the interventricular septum and terminates in the apex. The left bundle branch courses down the interventricular septum and divides into anterior and posterior fascicles before terminating in the apex. Electrical activity through the bundle branches is represented by the QRS complex. Refer to Chapter 7 to learn more about how to distinguish between these bundle branches on an EKG.

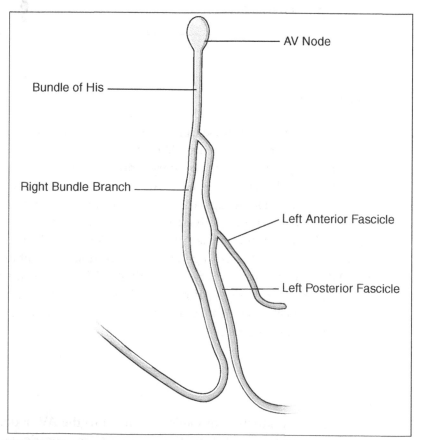

FIGURE 1.3

CHAPTER 1 REVIEW QUESTIONS

1. Normal sinus node activity occurs between _____ and _____ bpm.

2. If electricity spreads toward an area in the heart, the electrical impulse in the lead reflecting that area will be _____.

3. If electricity spreads away from an area in the heart, the electrical impulse in the lead reflecting that area will be _____.

4. All cardiac cells have a resting _____ charge.

5. The left bundle is composed of _____ and _____ fascicles.

6. The "gatekeeper" for electrical impulses through the heart is the _____.

7. The bundle branches are composed of rapidly conducting fibers called _____.

Defining the Intervals

INTRODUCTION

The various intervals seen on the EKG include:

- The P wave: represents atrial depolarization
- The QRS complex: represents ventricular depolarization
- The ST segment: represents the total ventricular repolarization time
- The T wave: represents the rapid phase of ventricular repolarization
- The QT interval: represents the entirety of ventricular systole

The classic 12-lead EKG represents about 6 seconds of time. On the EKG paper, one large box is equal to 200 milliseconds or 0.2 seconds. Each large box is composed of five smaller boxes, each equal to 40 milliseconds or 0.04 seconds. This is helpful to remember when estimating intervals (EKG 2.1).

The baseline of the EKG is defined as the isoelectric or flat line seen between the waveforms that comprise the P wave, QRS complex, and T wave. When considering segment elevation or depression, each small box represents 1 mm. You will hear ST segment elevation or depression described by the number of millimeters it is above or below the baseline.

The P wave, QRS complex, and T wave are individual components that together comprise important intervals that describe atrial and ventricular depolarization and repolarization (EKG 2.2).

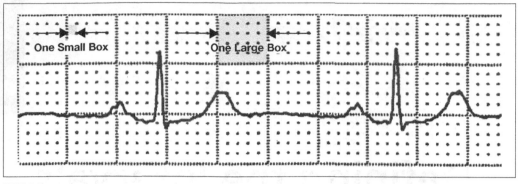

EKG 2.1

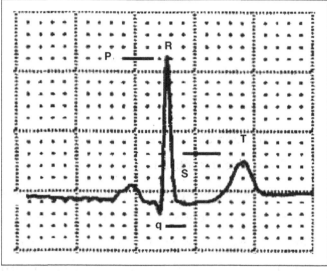

EKG 2.2

PR INTERVAL

The **PR interval** is the interval from the beginning of the P wave, which represents atrial depolarization, to the tip of the R wave, the elevated middle point of the QRS complex. The PR interval represents the time it takes for electricity to spread from the sinus node to the atrioventricular (AV) node. This interval represents the time necessary to allow for ventricular filling. A normal PR interval should fall between three and five small boxes or less than one large box on EKG. This represents 120 to 200 milliseconds or 0.12 to 0.2 seconds of time (EKG 2.3). If the PR interval is less than 0.12 seconds, this may indicate pre-excitation or early activation of the ventricles. This is seen in some forms of supraventricular tachycardia that involve bypass tracts. If the PR interval is greater than 0.2 seconds, this is consistent with first-degree AV block (EKG 2.4). This indicates that the conduction is taking longer than it should to spread from the sinus node to the AV node. *Clinical Point*: An additional clinical abnormality that can be seen with the PR interval is a depression of the PR interval below baseline. This is typically seen in pericarditis.

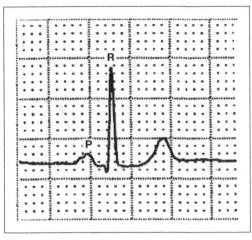

EKG 2.3

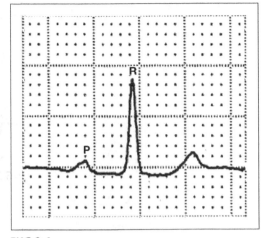

EKG 2.4

QRS DURATION

Normal **QRS duration** is 80 to 120 milliseconds or 0.08 to 0.12 seconds. This is equal to three small boxes or less on EKG (EKG 2.5). The QRS duration represents the depolarization of both the right and left ventricles. Any prolongation or widening of the QRS complex represents a delay in conduction through one or both of these bundle branches (EKG 2.6). More specifics of this conduction delay will be covered in Chapter 7. *Clinical Point*: A QRS duration greater than three small boxes indicates that there is a conduction delay somewhere in one or both ventricles.

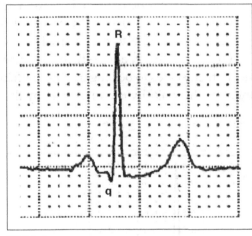

EKG 2.5

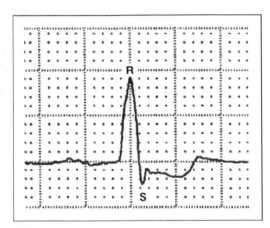

EKG 2.6

Because the QRS complex represents the pathway that electricity travels through the ventricles, there can be variations in its appearance. This may be due to areas of scar tissue, conduction delays, or normal variations. It is vital to understand the naming conventions used to describe the three components of the QRS complex (EKG 2.7). Not every ventricular complex has a Q wave, R wave, and S wave.

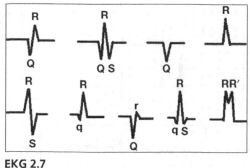

EKG 2.7

• Capital letters refer to larger deflections, greater than two small boxes.

• Lower case letters refer to smaller deflections, less than two small boxes.

• The Q wave is the first downward deflection.

• The R wave is the first upward deflection.

• The S wave is defined as the first negative deflection after an R wave.

• If there is more than one upward deflection, the second deflection is referred to as R prime (R′).

ST SEGMENT

The **ST segment** is the flat area of baseline situated between the QRS complex and T wave that represents the initial phase of ventricular repolarization, referred to as the plateau phase (EKG 2.8). It is the ventricles' answer to the PR interval. Just as there needs to be a delay to allow blood to fill from the atria to the ventricles (PR interval), there needs to be a delay that starts in the ventricles to allow them to return to an electrical steady state so that they can ready themselves to beat again. Ventricular repolarization is minimal during the ST segment, as the majority is represented by the T wave itself.

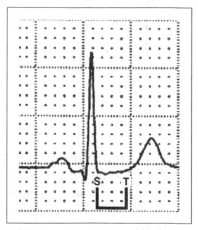

EKG 2.8

When examining the ST segment, be careful to look for the presence of ST segment elevation or depression. The ST segment should be isoelectric or flat on the baseline. *Clinical Point*: Deviation of 2 mm (two small boxes) above or below the baseline is indicative of a pathologic process.

The **J point** is where the QRS complex ends and the ST segment begins. J point elevation is a common and usually benign finding on EKG in younger patients. In classic ST segment elevation seen during an acute injury pattern, the ST segment is convex at the takeoff of the ST segment. If J point elevation is present, the ST segment will be concave. This finding is also referred to as early repolarization, but this concept is beyond the scope of this book. Compare J point elevation, ST segment elevation, and a normal EKG tracing side by side in EKGs 2.9 to 2.11, as this is an important clinical distinction to make.

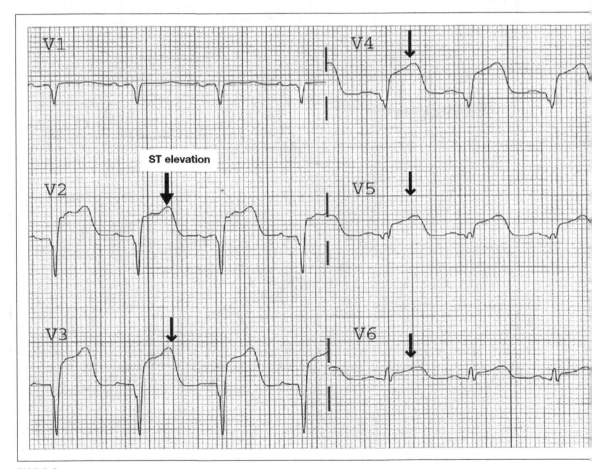

EKG 2.9

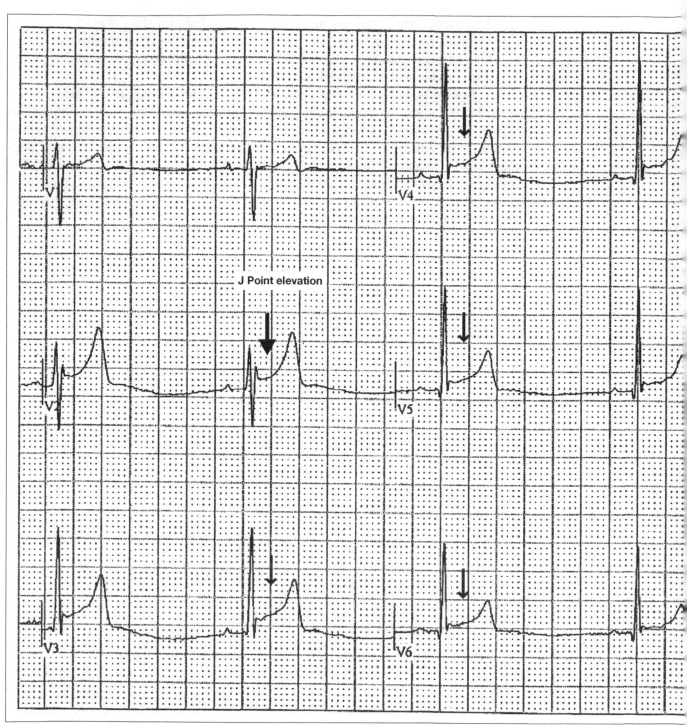

EKG 2.10

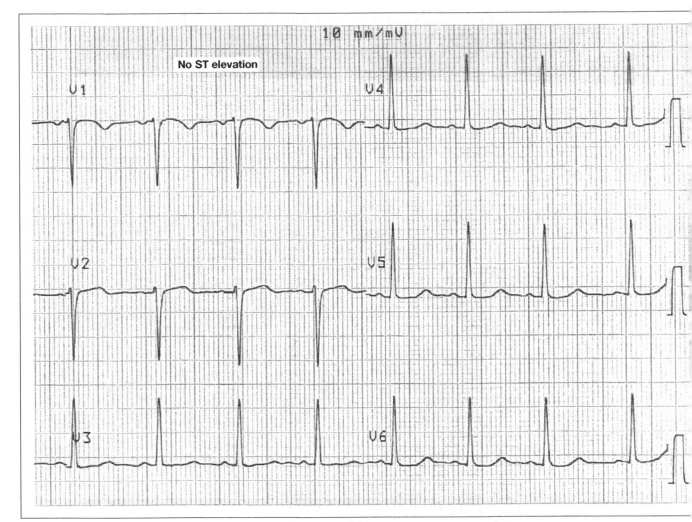

EKG 2.11

T WAVE

The **T wave** represents rapid ventricular repolarization. It is during this time that the myocytes regain their resting negative charge. The interval from the S wave to the apex of the T wave is termed the **absolute refractory period**. During this phase, the cells are essentially turned off to external stimuli. Once this period has passed, malignant ventricular arrhythmias can occur if the cellular milieu is unstable. For instance, ventricular arrhythmias can be initiated by a premature ventricular complex that falls after the apex of the T wave.

Two characteristics should be always noted with regard to the T wave: **inversion** and **peaked appearance**. Observe the morphology of the T wave in the normal tracing (EKG 2.12) and compare it with the abnormal T waves in EKGs 2.13 and 2.14. Inverted T waves may represent an old infarction or evolving ischemia. This is because scar tissue alters the route that electricity takes to spread through the heart, changing the appearance of the T wave (EKG 2.13). If the T wave is peaked, this represents electrical instability. *Clinical Point*: This is typically caused by electrolyte abnormalities, such as hyperkalemia (EKG 2.14).

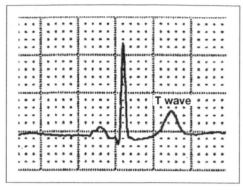

EKG 2.12

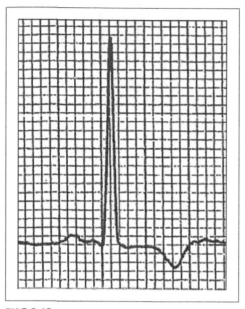

EKG 2.13

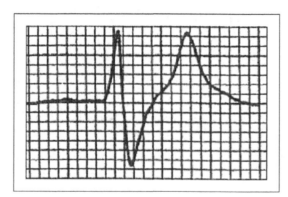

EKG 2.14

QT INTERVAL

This interval represents the entirety of ventricular systole. To accurately define the length of the interval, one must take into account the heart rate. This is called the corrected QT interval or **QTc**. As the heart rate increases, the R-R interval shortens, and therefore, the QT interval shortens. As the heart rate decreases, the R-R interval lengthens and the QT interval lengthens. The QT interval is always dependent on the heart rate.

It is imperative to accurately identify the end of the T wave. This can be difficult to do. Draw a slanted line from the peak of the T wave and continue down until it intersects the baseline. The distance from the Q wave to where the slanted line intersects the baseline is the QT interval (EKG 2.15).

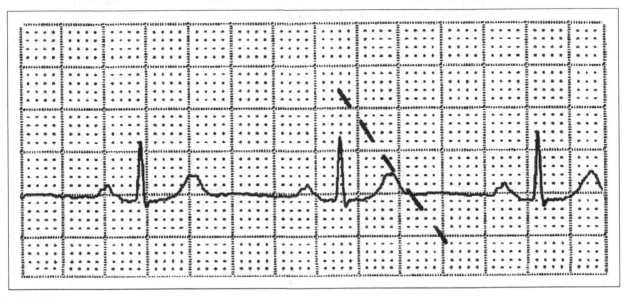

EKG 2.15

The actual formula to calculate the corrected QT interval is $QTc = QT/\sqrt{RR}$. An easy way to estimate this is to remember that the QTc should be less than half the R-R interval, using the R wave before and after the QT interval you are measuring. In general, the corrected QT interval should be between 340 and 460 milliseconds or 0.34 and 0.46 seconds. Any prolongation represents an instability in the ventricles' ability to effectively repolarize, increasing the risk of life-threatening ventricular arrhythmias.

Clinical Point: QT prolongation can be due to many causes, but it is frequently seen in electrolyte abnormalities such as hypokalemia. Certain medications can also prolong the QT interval, specifically antiarrhythmic medications due to their intended action to slow intracardiac ion channels. Certain antibiotics, antifungal medications, and some antipsychotics can also prolong the QTc. If a prolonged QTc is present, the patient's medication list should be closely examined. Concomitant use of the above-mentioned medications can be a recipe for disaster.

U WAVE

The **U wave** is a diastolic deflection sometimes seen at the end of the T wave (EKG 2.16). The junction of the T and U waves should be isoelectric or situated along the baseline. *Clinical Point*: The presence of an upright U wave is generally considered a normal variant; however, it can be more prominent in the setting of hypokalemia and left ventricular volume overload. A U wave is much more likely to be present when the heart rate is less than 65 bpm and is almost never seen when the heart rate is more than 95 bpm, as it is usually buried in the T wave.

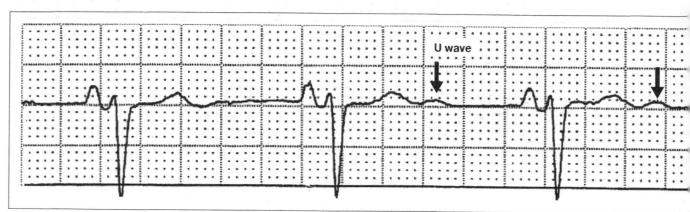

EKG 2.16

CHAPTER 2 REVIEW QUESTIONS

1. A normal PR interval is _____.

2. A normal QRS duration is _____.

3. A normal QT interval is _____.

4. QTc prolongation can lead to _____.

5. Which interval represents the entirety of ventricular systole?

6. The end of the QRS and beginning of the ST segment is referred to as the _____.

7. Is a U wave more likely to be seen during tachycardia or bradycardia?

8. Which part of the EKG marks the end of the absolute refractory period?

Lead Review

INTRODUCTION

A 12-lead EKG provides a wealth of information once we know what and where to look for it and how to interpret what we find.

The human body conducts electricity. By placing electrodes at varying but consistent distances from the heart, the flow of electrical currents can be measured from the heart to those points. This provides a wealth of information regarding the location of heart block, ischemia, and infarction by creating electrical vectors that comprise the standard 12-lead EKG.

TYPES AND PLACEMENT OF LEADS

There are two types of leads: **limb leads** and **chest leads**. Review Figure 3.1 for limb lead placement. Review Figure 3.2 for chest lead placement.

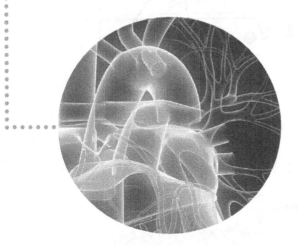

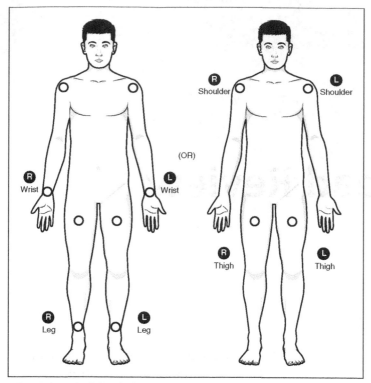

FIGURE 3.1 Limb lead placement.

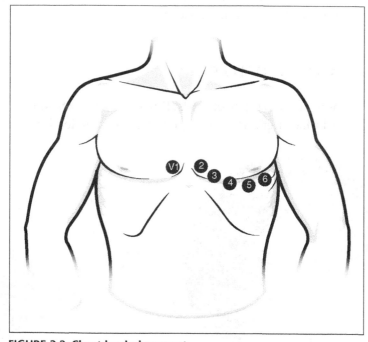

FIGURE 3.2 Chest lead placement.

LIMB LEADS

The limb leads are the leads that are used to define the cardiac axis (EKG 3.1). There are two types of limb leads:

- **Bipolar leads**

  Leads I, II, and III

- **Unipolar augmented leads**

  Leads aVR, aVL, and aVF

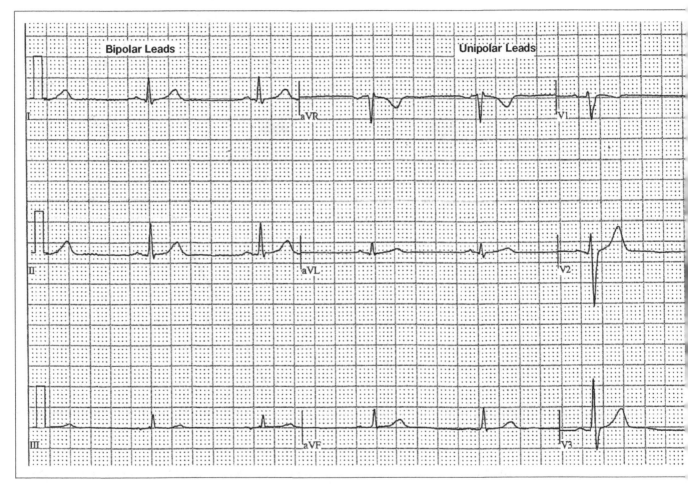

EKG 3.1

Bipolar Limb Leads

Leads I, II, and **III** are the standard limb leads. They are bipolar, meaning they have a positive pole and a negative pole. These leads record electrical voltages in one position relative to another position using the left arm electrode (LA), the right arm electrode (RA), and the left leg electrode (LL). The right leg electrode functions as an electrical grounding system (Figure 3.3).

- Lead I records the electrical difference between the left arm and the right arm electrodes and is positive on the left and negative on the right

- Lead II records the electrical difference between the left leg and the right arm electrodes and is positive at the leg and negative at the arm

- Lead III records the electrical difference between the left leg and the left arm electrodes and is positive at the leg and negative at the arm

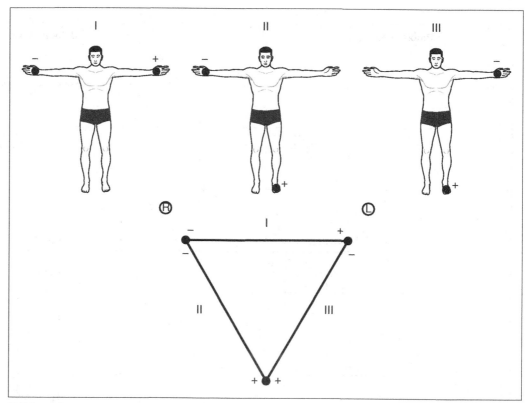

FIGURE 3.3

By measuring the electrical difference between these leads relative to each other, vectors or angles are created through the heart, which we can see on an EKG. These leads were designed to represent three sides of an equilateral triangle with the heart residing in the center. Together, these three leads comprise **Einthoven's triangle**, named after the Dutch physician whom most consider the father of the modern EKG (Figure 3.4).

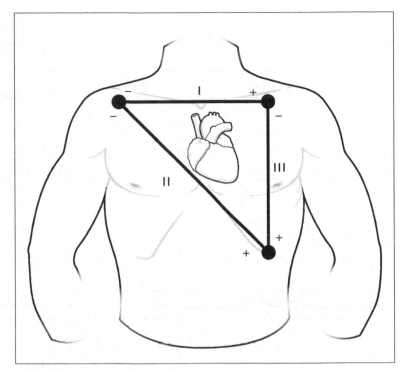

FIGURE 3.4 Einthoven's triangle.

Einthoven's law states that the magnitude of the deflection of lead II is equal to the sum of the deflections of leads I and III. **Einthoven's equation** states that **I + III = II**. Considering Einthoven's triangle, the left arm is positive in lead I and negative in lead III and, therefore, these leads cancel each other out when added together. As a result of the combination of all three sides of the triangle (I, II, and III), there is one single vector (lead II) that represents the sum of the electromotive forces of the heart. In any given EKG, the voltage of lead I plus the voltage of lead III should equal the voltage in lead II. If it does not, this should raise suspicion of lead misplacement. Refer to EKG 3.2 for this point.

Count the number of small boxes in each QRS complex to calculate voltage.

- QRS in lead I = 5 small boxes
- QRS in lead II = 8 small boxes
- QRS in lead III = 3 small boxes

Calculate: Lead I (5) + Lead III (3) = Lead II (8). The lead placement in this example is accurate.

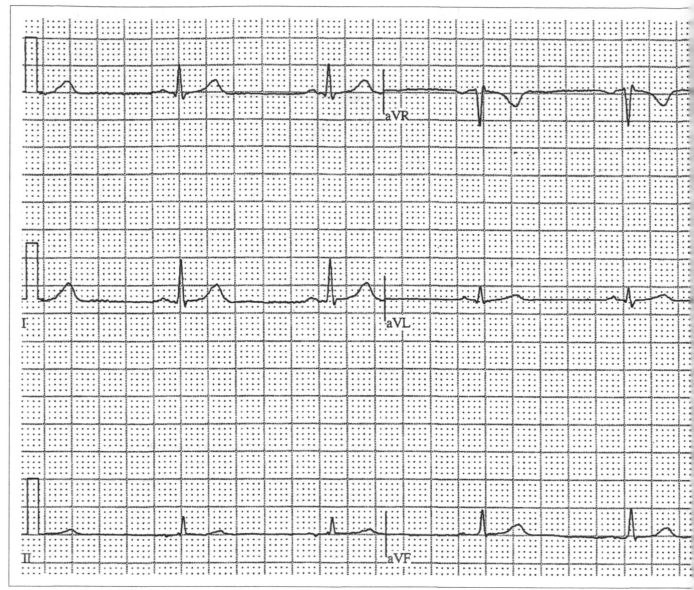

EKG 3.2

Unipolar Augmented Leads

If an intersecting line is drawn through each of the angles created by Einthoven's triangle, several new vectors are created through which to view electrical activity within the heart (Figure 3.5). This results in the creation of the three unipolar augmented leads **aVR**, **aVL**, and **aVF**.

- aVR: Augmented voltage right arm: a combination of leads I and II
- aVL: Augmented voltage left arm: a combination of leads I and III
- aVF: Augmented voltage foot: a combination of leads II and III

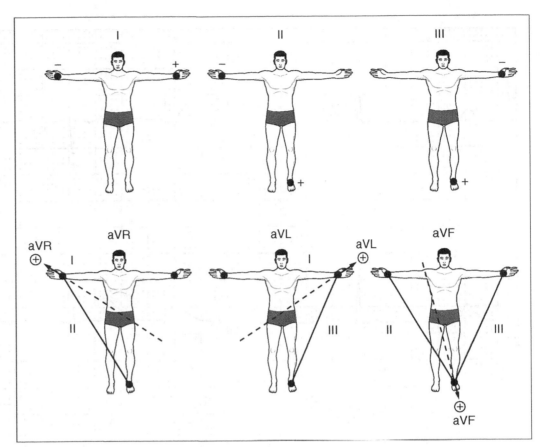

FIGURE 3.5

In contrast to the bipolar leads, the unipolar leads record voltages at one location relative to zero rather than relative to another lead.

The locations of the electrodes which comprise these leads are not in close proximity to the heart. In order to be more readable, aVR, aVL, and aVF are augmented over the actual voltage from each extremity, hence the term "augmented leads". When added together, the QRS voltage in each unipolar lead should equal 0. Refer to EKG 3.3 for an illustration of this point.

Count the number of small boxes in each QRS complex to calculate voltage:

- QRS voltage in lead aVR = −7

- QRS voltage in lead aVL = +3

- QRS voltage in lead aVF = +4

    Calculate: aVR (−7) + aVL (3) + aVF (4) = 0

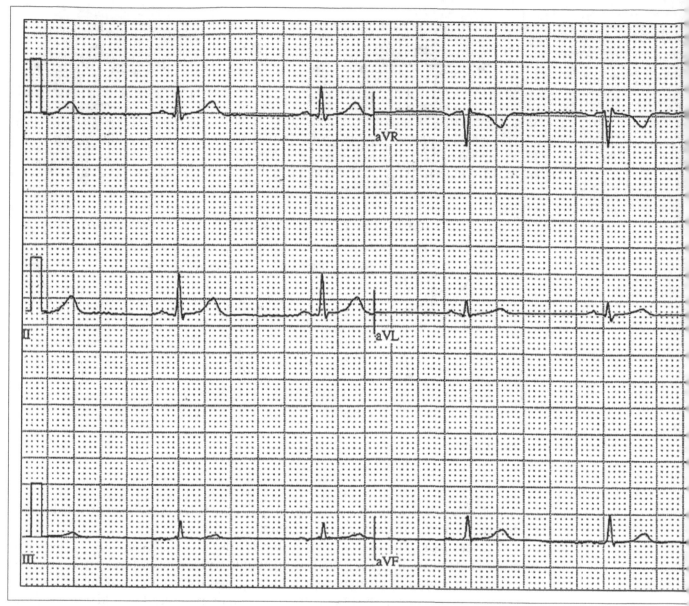

EKG 3.3

REVIEW OF IMPORTANT POINTS

Bipolar leads: Contain a positive and a negative pole

- Lead I is a horizontal line across the body and is negative at the right arm and positive at the left arm.

- Lead II is a diagonal line that is positive at the left foot and negative at the right arm.

- Lead III is a diagonal line that is positive at the left foot and negative at the left arm.
- **I + III = II**

Unipolar augmented leads: Contain only a positive pole:

- aVR: Augmented voltage right arm: a combination of leads I and II
- aVL: Augmented voltage left arm: a combination of leads I and III
- aVF: Augmented voltage foot: a combination of leads II and III
- **aVR + aVL + aVF = 0**

COMBINING UNIPOLAR AND BIPOLAR LEADS

By using all of the unipolar and bipolar leads together, significantly more angles are created from which see the heart's electrical activity. Using the knowledge about the origin of these leads, a helpful picture can be drawn starting with Einthoven's triangle (Figure 3.6).

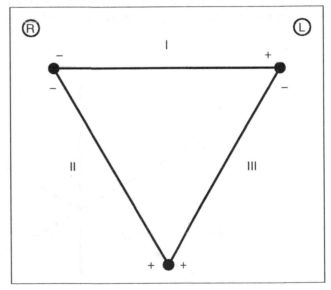

FIGURE 3.6

Shift the leads in this triangle so that they intersect at a common central point (Figure 3.7).

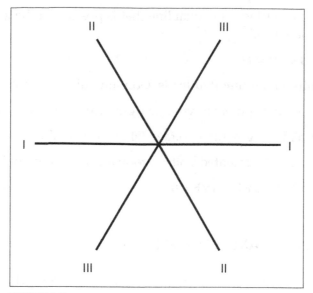

FIGURE 3.7

Create a second diagram by shifting the augmented leads to intersect at a common central point. Recall that aVR is directed toward the right arm, aVL is directed toward the left arm, and aVF is directed toward the feet (Figure 3.8).

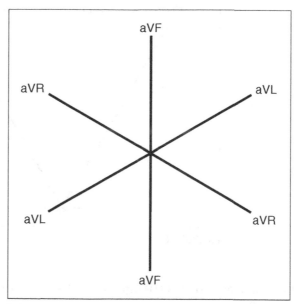

FIGURE 3.8

Combine these two together to create a diagram that shows the exact relationship between the bipolar leads and the unipolar leads (Figure 3.9). It is this relationship that defines the cardiac axis. All of this information will be applied in Chapter 6 when discussing how to determine the electrical axis of the EKG.

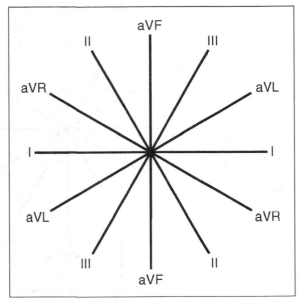

FIGURE 3.9

Each of these leads records the same electrical activity, but from a different angle. This is why the EKG tracing will vary from lead to lead. As depolarization spreads toward a positive pole, there is an upward deflection in that lead. As it spreads away from a positive pole, there is a downward deflection in that lead. Take the vantage point of each positive pole. As electricity moves toward it, the respective EKG deflection appears positive. As electricity moves away from it, it appears negative (Figure 3.10).

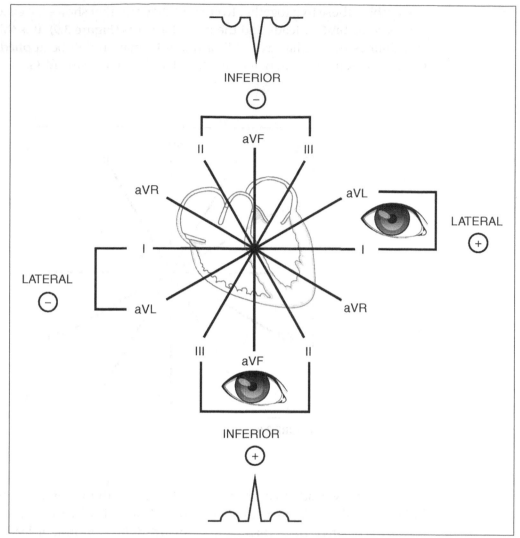

FIGURE 3.10

PLACEMENT OF THE CHEST LEADS

The chest leads are leads V1 to V6. These are also referred to as precordial leads because they are placed directly over the chest wall in close proximity to the heart. Similar to the augmented leads, the precordial leads only have a positive pole. They also use a central terminal, or V lead, for their negative pole. These leads do not figure into axis determination.

Chest lead placement is as follows (Figures 3.11 and 3.12):

• V1: Right fourth intercostal space

• V2: Left fourth intercostal space

- V3: On the left, directly in between V2 and V4

- V4: Left fifth intercostal space in the midclavicular line

- V5: Even with V4 in the anterior axillary line

- V6: Even with V4 and V5 in the midaxillary line

  - In women, leads V3 to V6 should be placed just under the breast tissue, but still in the appropriate anatomical line.

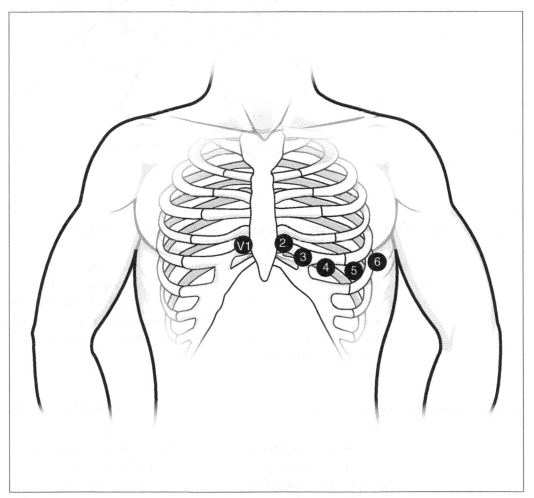

FIGURE 3.11

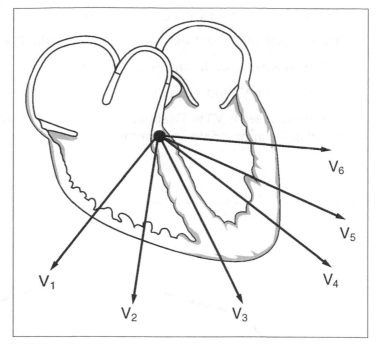

FIGURE 3.12

BASIC INTERPRETATION OF THE QRS COMPLEX ACROSS THE PRECORDIAL LEADS

Considering the QRS complexes in the precordial leads, the R waves should become taller and the S wave smaller as you move from right to left. In V1 and V2, there should be a deep S wave. Usually around lead V3, the R wave and S wave will be of equal height. There should be a complete transition by lead V4, where the R wave should be distinctly larger or the QRS more positive by this point, and remain so as you continue over to lead V6.

R WAVE PROGRESSION

The term **R wave progression** refers to these normal changes that occur in the QRS complex as you move across the chest leads. Poor R wave progression refers to nonadherence to these rules and is rather nonspecific. Anything that changes the depolarization of either ventricle will change this progression. Common causes of this include right or left ventricular hypertrophy, a left anterior fascicular block, and infarction. These will be specifically addressed in Chapters 6 to 8. Compare the appearance of normal R wave progression (EKG 3.4) to a lack of R wave progression (EKG 3.5) across the precordial leads.

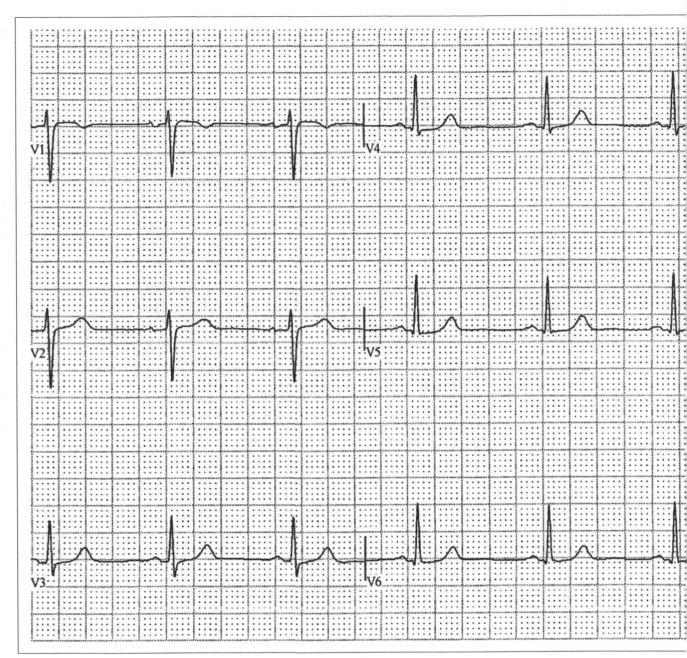

EKG 3.4

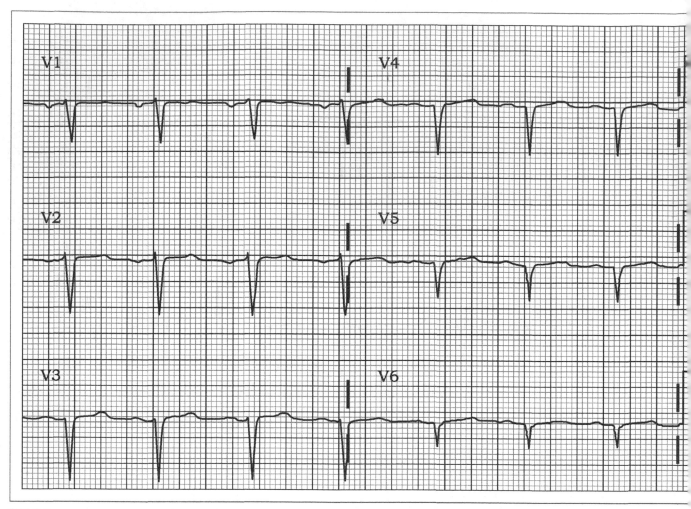

EKG 3.5

APPLYING THE GROUP PATTERN OF 12-LEAD EKG INTERPRETATION

These 12 leads should be always considered in groups because each set of leads represents a specific area of the myocardium (EKG 3.6). Following a pattern is essential to correctly and efficiently interpret EKGs. Leads I, aVL, V5, and V6 are the lateral leads. Leads II, III, and aVF are the inferior leads. Leads V1 to V4 are the anterior chest leads. Leads V1 and V2 are more specifically referred to as anteroseptal leads. Lead aVR does not offer a direct view of the left ventricle and therefore does not fit into any of these groups. It represents the area of the right ventricular outflow tract and basal interventricular septum. It is an important lead to consider when determining the origin of atrial and ventricular arrhythmias, but that is beyond the scope of this book.

- Lateral: I, aVL, V5, V6

- Inferior: II, III, aVF

- Anterior: V1 to V4

  ◦ Anteroseptal: V1 to V2

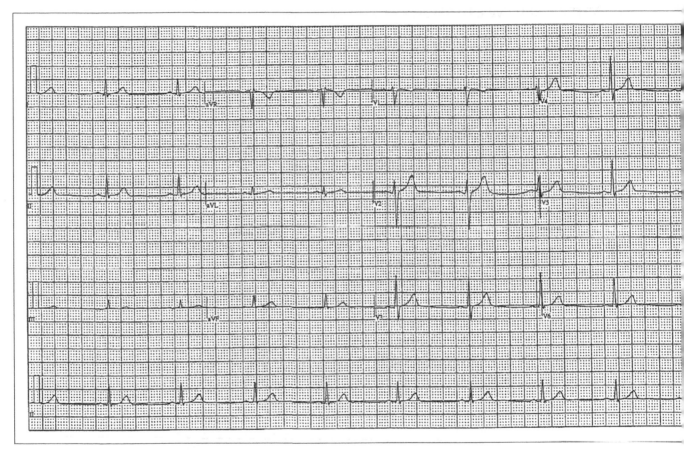

EKG 3.6

CHAPTER 3 REVIEW QUESTIONS

1. Which leads are bipolar?

2. Which leads are unipolar?

3. aVF is a combination of which leads?

4. aVL is a combination of which leads?

5. aVR is a combination of which leads?

6. As depolarization spreads toward a positive pole, there is a _____ deflection in that lead.

7. As depolarization spreads away from a positive pole, there is a _____ deflection in that lead.

8. The R wave should be distinctly larger than the S wave by which precordial lead?

Rate

It is imperative to implement a systematic approach to EKG interpretation. There are five main areas to master. They are rate, rhythm, axis, block, and infarction. If you review each EKG and identify and appropriately interpret these five areas, you will know everything you need to know about that EKG.

CALCULATING THE HEART RATE

The standard calculation used to convey heart rate is beats per minute (bpm). A normal heart rate that originates in the sinus node is 60 to 100 bpm. Recall that the term automaticity refers to areas of the heart that have the ability to initiate a pacemaker impulse. Every cell in the heart is capable of initiating an action potential and stimulating the heart to beat, but only a few areas do this on a routine basis. These areas of cells, or foci, are found in **the sinus node, the atrioventricular node**, and in **the ventricles** (Figure 4.1). Each area of automaticity carries a different intrinsic heart rate. All these areas are capable of initiating a cardiac impulse, but the fastest pacemaker always wins and sets the pace for the rest of the conduction system to follow.

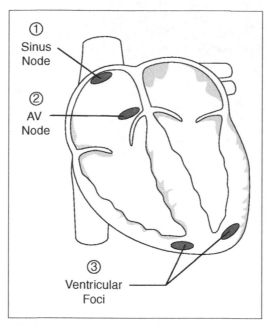

FIGURE 4.1

By design, the fastest focus is the sinus node. It has an intrinsic rate of 60 to 100 bpm. The atrioventricular node has an intrinsic rate of 40 to 60 bpm. The ventricles trigger impulses at 20 to 40 bpm. *Clinical Point*: The lower in the conduction system the focus is located, the more unstable and unreliable it is.

All slower foci are overdrive suppressed by their faster counterparts. If an automaticity area fails to generate an impulse in a timely fashion, the next fastest pacemaker will become the dominant one and set the pace. By definition, impulses that are generated from the atrioventricular node and the ventricles will not have a P wave in front of them, because a P wave represents sinus node activity. The overdrive suppression order, or a chain of command within the heart, is seen in Table 4.1.

TABLE 4.1 Overdrive Suppression Order

Automaticity Area	P Wave	QRS Duration	Rate (bpm)
Sinus node	Present	Normal	60–100
AV node	Absent	Normal or slightly prolonged	40–60
Ventricle	Absent	Very prolonged	20–40

Recall that a low atrial focus is represented by inverted P waves. This stimulus originates from somewhere in between the sinus node and the atrioventricular node. The heart rate is reflected as such.

In determining rate, P waves can be ignored for now. Calculate the heart rate by looking at the R waves. Identify an R wave that falls on one of the thick black lines that comprises one large box. Count 300, 150, 100, 75, 60, 50, 40 for each large box that comes after this until arriving at the next R wave (EKG 4.1). The heart rate is calculated with ease if the next R wave falls on a thick black line. If it does not, the heart rate can be accurately estimated as it will fall in between two of those numbers. Using this simple method, the heart rate in EKG 4.1 can be determined to be approximately 65 bpm.

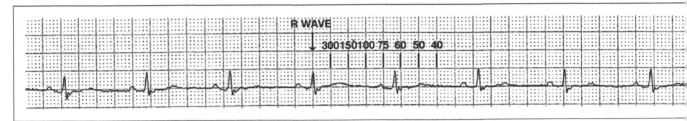

EKG 4.1

If the calculated heart rate is between 60 and 100 bpm and there is a normal, upright P wave before each QRS, the automaticity focus generating that impulse is within the sinus node. Heart rates greater than 100 bpm that have a normal appearing P wave before them are still (usually) sinus in origin. This is consistent with sinus tachycardia (EKG 4.2).

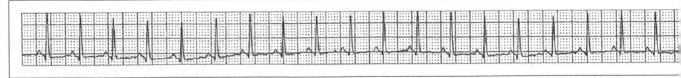

EKG 4.2

If the impulse is less than 60 bpm but there is still a P wave before every QRS, this is consistent with sinus bradycardia. The presence of a P wave defines its origin within the sinus node (EKG 4.3).

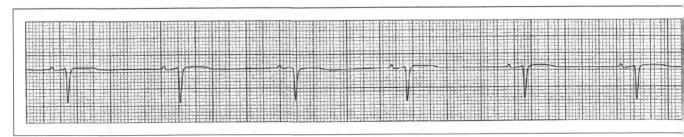

EKG 4.3

This method of quickly calculating heart rate does not work for rates less than 40 bpm. Most EKGs have 3-second markers on them. If not, the EKG can be divided into two parts as the typical EKG is 6 seconds long. Count how many QRS complexes there are in a 6-second rhythm strip, printed along the bottom of most EKGs. This number can be divided by 2, multiplied by 10, and results in an accurate estimation of the heart rate. This is also an effective method when there is an irregular rhythm. This method can be applied to EKG 4.4. There are six QRS complexes in the 6-second rhythm strip. Six divided by two is three. Three times 10 is 30 bpm.

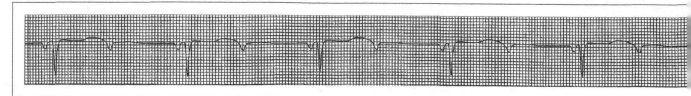

EKG 4.4

JUNCTIONAL RHYTHMS

Anything that originates below the sinus node is called a **junctional rhythm**. If the heart rate is 40 to 60 bpm and there is no P wave before each QRS, the impulse is being generated from the atrioventricular node (EKG 4.5). If the heart rate is 20 to 40 bpm and there is no P wave before each QRS, the impulse is being generated from the ventricles (EKG 4.6). Recall that by definition, an AV nodal junctional focus will have a narrow or only slightly prolonged QRS, while a ventricular focus will be very wide.

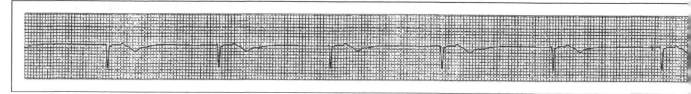

EKG 4.5

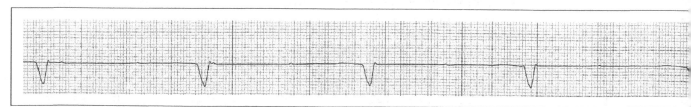

EKG 4.6

In EKG 4.7, a ventricular escape rhythm gradually transitions to and from normal sinus rhythm. Note the initial lack of P waves prior to a wide QRS followed by the appearance of P waves and a narrowing of the QRS.

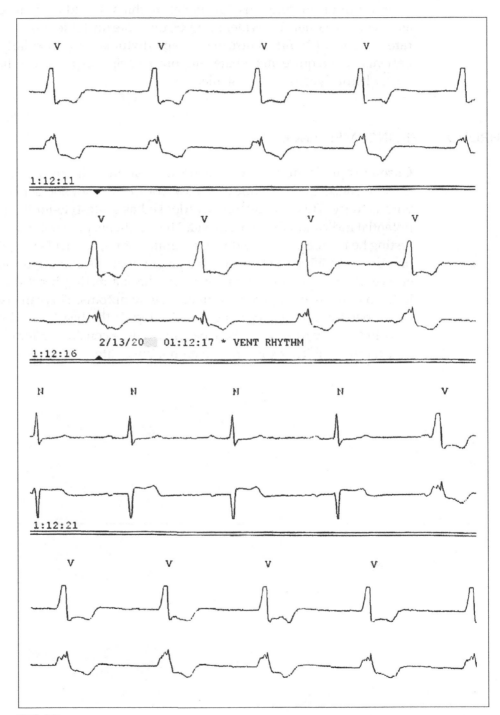

EKG 4.7

Junctional rhythms are frequently associated with overmedication. They can also be seen in fibrocalcific conduction disease, or the normal aging process of the conduction system. Always closely examine the patient's medication list for rate-slowing medications, such as beta blockers, calcium channel blockers, digoxin, and antiarrhythmic medications. Junctional rhythms should be defined by their origin, as described earlier. The wider the QRS, the more unstable and unreliable the escape rate is. *Clinical Point*: Ventricular escape rhythms are particularly unstable. These patients may require immediate temporary pacing, especially if they are symptomatic or hemodynamically unstable.

CHRONOTROPIC INCOMPETENCE

Chronotropic incompetence is defined by an inability of the sinus node to effectively increase the sinus rate and allow for the physiologic demand that is present with activity. This is frequently overlooked as a lifestyle-limiting condition and a potential indication for a pacemaker. These patients may not have dangerously low resting heart rates, but they do have significant impairments in their ability to carry on normal activities. Patients will complain of persistent fatigue and exercise intolerance. If they are already on telemetry, check a resting heart rate and walk them in the hall in an attempt to reproduce their symptoms. This can also be determined by outpatient ambulatory holter monitoring. If the heart rate does not appropriately increase with activity, these patients may be considered for permanent pacing, which can significantly improve their quality of life.

CHAPTER 4 REVIEW QUESTIONS

1. Normal sinus activity occurs at rates between _____ and _____ bpm.

2. An AV nodal junctional focus will fire at a rate between _____ and _____ bpm.

3. Ventricular escape focus will fire between _____ and _____ bpm.

4. Calculate the heart rate of the patient in the 6-second rhythm strip below. Is it originating from the sinus node, AV node, or in the ventricles?

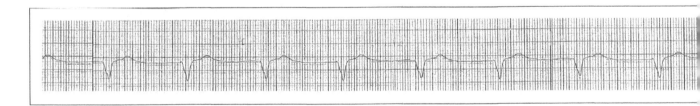

5. Calculate the heart rate of the patient in the 6-second rhythm strip below. Is it originating from the sinus node, AV node, or in the ventricles?

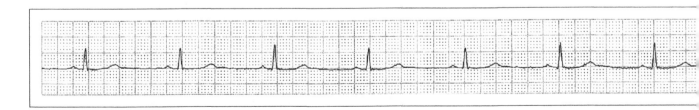

Rhythm

INTRODUCTION

The next critical point to master after calculating the heart rate is the evaluation of the rhythm. This can be done by establishing the presence or absence of regularly occurring QRS complexes. Simply put, evaluate if the rhythm is regular or irregular. Using calipers, march from R wave to R wave across the EKG. If the QRS complexes march out at even intervals all the way across the page, the rhythm is regular (EKG 5.1). If there is a variation, the rhythm is irregular (EKG 5.2). An irregular rhythm is not necessarily pathologic. This chapter will focus on how to identify irregular rhythms and further classify them as normal or abnormal. If a rhythm is identified as irregular, it must be further classified as regularly irregular or irregularly irregular. These points are accomplished by properly identifying the presence or absence of patterns and evaluating the P wave.

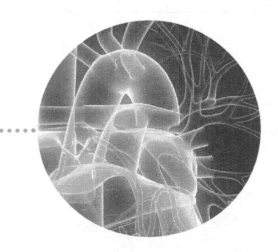

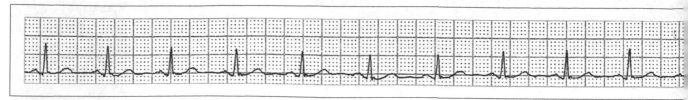

EKG 5.1

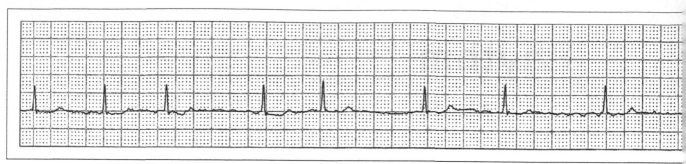

EKG 5.2

THE AUTONOMIC NERVOUS SYSTEM AND HEART RATE VARIATION

Regularly irregular rhythms follow a pattern and can be physiologically normal. This is because the autonomic nervous system plays a vital role in normal heart rate variation (Figure 5.1).

The following are the important points to remember:

• The vagus nerve innervates the sinus node and the atrioventricular (AV) node.

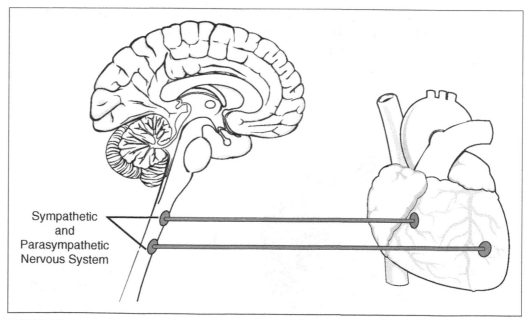

Sympathetic and Parasympathetic Nervous System

FIGURE 5.1

- Sympathetic stimulation decreases vagal tone. This causes the sinus node to speed up, which is seen on EKG as sinus tachycardia in a fight-or-flight response (Figure 5.2).
- Parasympathetic stimulation increases vagal tone. This allows for slow resting heart rates during relaxation (Figure 5.2).
- On EKG, increased vagal tone and parasympathetic stimulation can appear as sinus bradycardia, sinus pauses, or AV block.
- The vagus nerve also innervates the stomach. An increased vagal tone can be seen in the setting of nausea and vomiting.

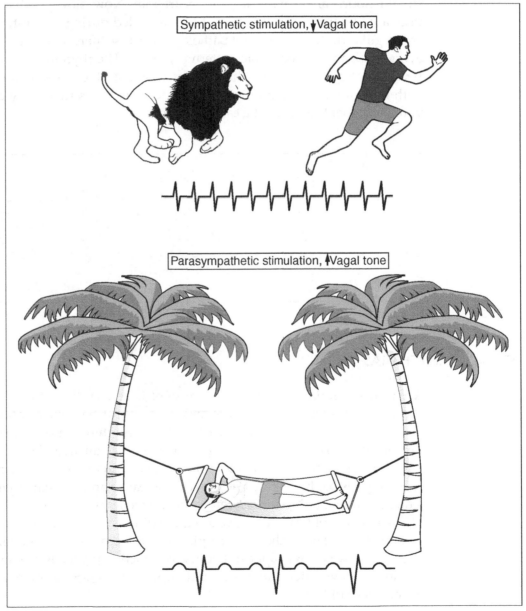

FIGURE 5.2

SINUS ARRHYTHMIA

The autonomic nervous system is constantly active within the cardiovascular system. One of the most common and nonpathologic irregular rhythms seen in everyday practice is **sinus arrhythmia**. The most common cause of sinus arrhythmia is normal respiration. There is a slight increase in heart rate with inspiration and a slight decrease in heart rate with expiration (EKG 5.3). This is driven by the autonomic nervous system. It is a normal physiologic occurrence that allows for increased venous return and diastolic filling during inspiration.

Perform a "self-test." Palpate your radial pulse and take a deep breath in. You should notice an increase in your heart rate. Now slowly exhale and notice a decrease in your heart rate. If an EKG is recorded during this test, it would reveal an irregular rhythm. This is not pathologic, because there should be a P wave before every QRS, and a predictable pattern is present. The rhythm is regularly irregular. If you print out a longer rhythm strip, you will be able to see a pattern correlating with inspiration and expiration. Heart rate variation is frequently documented in younger patients and is not a cause for concern.

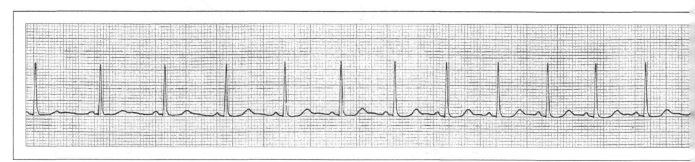

EKG 5.3

ATRIAL ARRHYTHMIAS

Atrial arrhythmias are a common cause of irregular rhythms, which are seen in clinical practice. Although most of these warrant further investigation, we can look at them on a continuum from least concerning rhythm to most. Begin with **premature atrial contractions** (PACs). A PAC occurs when an area of excitable cells in the atrium triggers conduction before the normal sinus node (Figure 5.3). A P wave is usually visible before the QRS. PACs will cause an irregular rhythm, but rarely require treatment unless it is for symptomatic relief (EKG 5.4).

The P waves of PACs will have a slightly different morphology from the P waves of sinus beats. The farther the ectopic focus is from the sinus node, the more different the P waves will appear. Because conduction proceeds as usual through the AV node and ventricles after the atrial impulse, the QRS duration is unchanged in the presence of PACs.

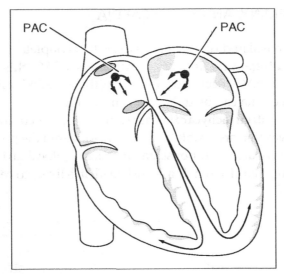

FIGURE 5.3

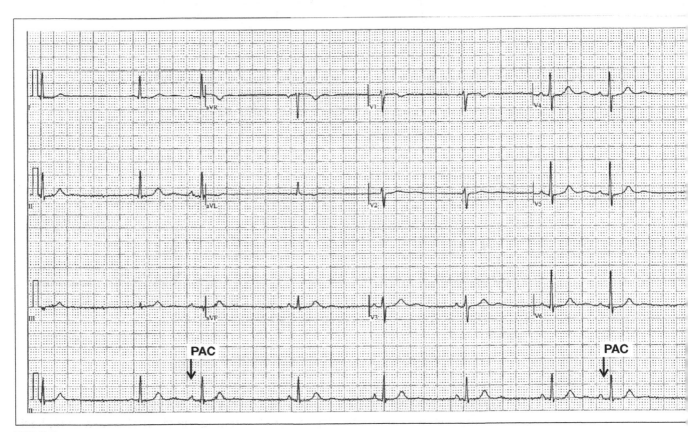

EKG 5.4

ATRIAL BIGEMINY, TRIGEMINY, AND TACHYCARDIA

PACs can be isolated or occur in pairs, called couplets. If every other beat is a PAC, this is **atrial bigeminy**. If every third beat is a PAC, this is **atrial trigeminy**. When three or more PACs occur consecutively, this is called **atrial tachycardia** (EKG 5.5). Atrial tachycardia can be unifocal or multifocal.

In **unifocal atrial tachycardia**, there is one ectopic focus initiating a rapid impulse. All of the P waves that are visible and not buried within the preceding T wave will appear the same. If occurring in nonsustained runs, unifocal atrial tachycardia will cause a regularly irregular rhythm. If it is sustained, it is likely to cause a regular rhythm.

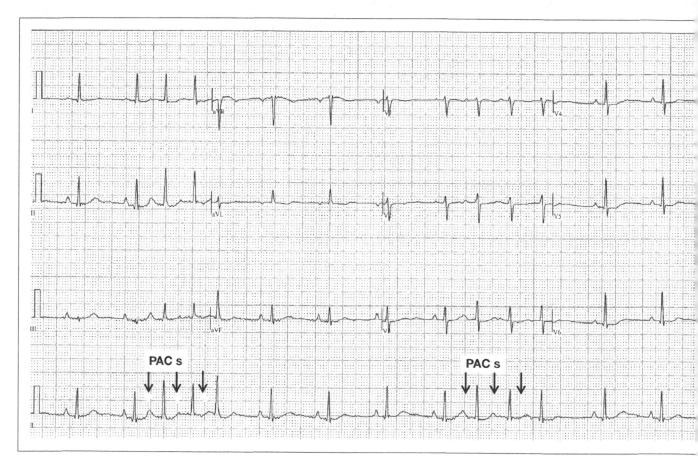

EKG 5.5

Multifocal atrial tachycardia is more likely to cause a slightly irregular rhythm because there is more than one atrial focus stimulating the ventricles (EKG 5.6). Each focus will have a slightly different automaticity, or intrinsic rate, and a slightly different morphology. When there is a beat-to-beat variance in P wave morphology at slower rates, this is referred to as a **wandering atrial pacemaker** and is usually associated with a regular rhythm. *Clinical Point*: Multifocal atrial tachycardia and a wandering atrial pacemaker are commonly associated with chronic and acute pulmonary conditions, such as COPD exacerbation.

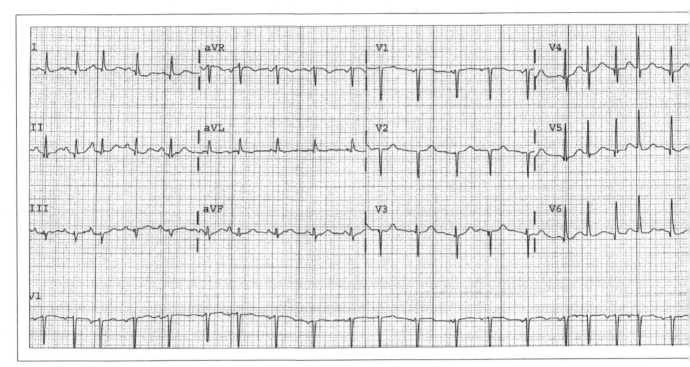

EKG 5.6

ATRIAL FIBRILLATION

Either type of atrial tachycardia can degenerate to a disorganized irregularly irregular rhythm called **atrial fibrillation**. Atrial fibrillation is the classic irregularly irregular arrhythmia. Recall from Chapter 1 that every cell in the heart is capable of initiating an action potential and causing the heart to beat. Usually, there is one dominant pacemaker, the sinus node. In atrial fibrillation, the cells in the atria are so electrically chaotic that no one focus is able to be the dominant pacemaker and initiate the electrical cascade. This results in disorganized, rapid stimulation of the atrial tissue, which then bombards the AV node with impulses at 300 bpm. Thankfully, the AV node will not allow this kind of conduction due to principles of refractoriness. After allowing one impulse to conduct (depolarizing), it must return to an electrical steady state (repolarize) before it can accept another. This prevents the ventricular rate from becoming excessively fast. The end result of this chaotic electrical activity is seen on an EKG as an irregularly irregular pattern of QRS complexes without any identifiable P waves (EKG 5.7). Atrial fibrillation will be discussed in further detail in Chapter 9.

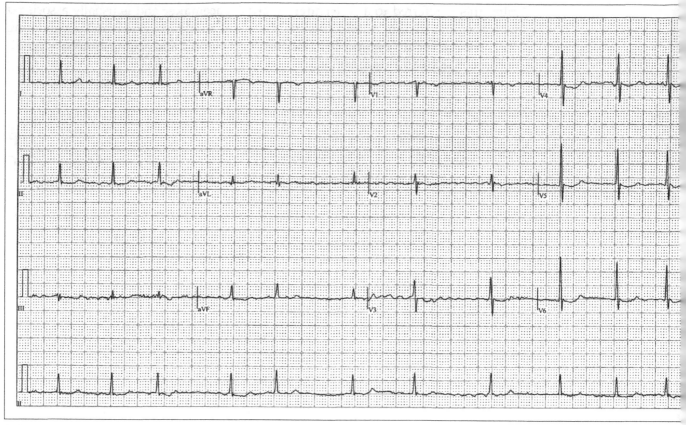

EKG 5.7

SUMARY OF ATRIAL ARRHYTHMIAS

- PACs can be isolated or occur in pairs.
- Three or more consecutive PACs are termed atrial tachycardia.
- Sustained atrial tachycardia will cause a regular rhythm.
- Nonsustained atrial tachycardia will cause a regularly irregular rhythm.
- Multifocal atrial tachycardia is more likely to be slightly irregular, and the P waves will all have a slightly different morphology from one another.
- Atrial tachycardia can further degenerate to atrial fibrillation, which is always an irregularly irregular rhythm.
- Atrial flutter is a more organized form of atrial fibrillation that is reviewed in detail in Chapter 9. It can cause a regular or an irregular pattern, depending on the atrial circuit conduction through the AV node.
- If a rhythm is identified as irregular, it must be further classified as regularly irregular or irregularly irregular. This is done simply by identifying the presence or absence of patterns, as discussed earlier.

VENTRICULAR ARRHYTHMIAS

Premature beats can also arise from the ventricle. These are called **premature ventricular contractions** (PVCs) and follow the same principles as PACs in terms of irregularity. Note the distinctly different appearance of a PVC from a sinus beat (EKG 5.8). This occurs because the electrical impulse is originating from an entirely different location than normal sinus node activation. These foci are areas of excitable tissue in the ventricles that initiate an impulse irregularly and erratically. PVCs are also commonly benign, particularly if they are unifocal and isolated. Multifocal PVCs have a differing appearance from one another and are more commonly associated with underlying structural heart disease. PVCs indicate that there is some degree of irritability in the ventricles, and it is up to the clinician to determine whether it is serious or benign. See Chapter 10 for more details regarding PVCs.

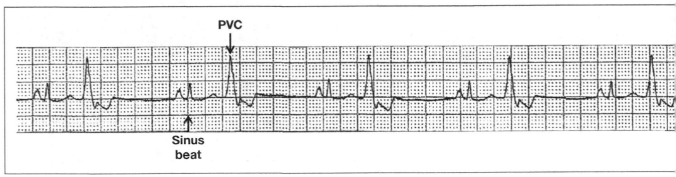

EKG 5.8

CHAPTER 5 REVIEW QUESTIONS

1. Is the below rhythm regular or irregular?

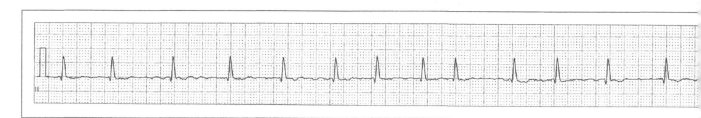

2. Is this rhythm regular or irregular?

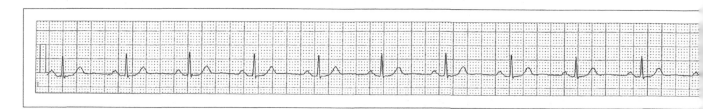

3. Atrial fibrillation will cause a(n) _____ rhythm with lack of clear _____.

4. Which results in more frequent PACs: atrial bigeminy or atrial trigeminy?

5. Will increased vagal tone cause the heart rate to increase or decrease?

Axis

INTRODUCTION

Axis refers to the general direction of electrical conduction through the heart. The QRS complex represents ventricular depolarization. Each lead represents a different angle, or vector of depolarization through the ventricular myocardium. All of these added together represent one average QRS vector, referred to as the axis.

Each patient will fall into one of four axis categories: **normal, left, right, or indeterminate**. This is determined based on the four quadrants that are created by the intersection of leads I and aVF. These two leads are the most important in determining axis. They intersect at the center of the heart and form four right angles. The normal vector points down and to the patient's left (Figures 6.1 and 6.2).

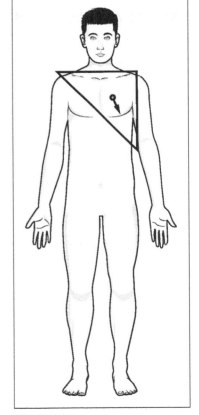

FIGURE 6.1

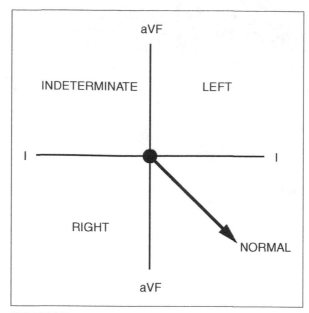

FIGURE 6.2

USING LIMB LEADS TO DEFINE AXIS IN DEGREES

Axis is described in degrees. Lead I runs from 0 to 180 degrees from the left arm to the right arm. Lead aVF runs from head to toe and therefore forms a right angle with lead I. The top and bottom of aVF can be labeled with 90 degrees (Figure 6.3). The resulting figure demonstrates the four quadrants: normal, left, right, and indeterminate.

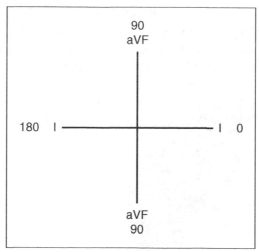

FIGURE 6.3

Leads II and III have to intersect lead I at a common central point and run in opposite directions. Lead II runs from 60 to 120 degrees, terminating at the left foot. Lead III runs from 60 to 120 degrees, terminating at the right foot (Figure 6.4).

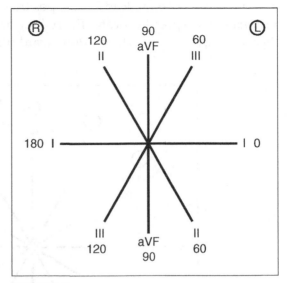

FIGURE 6.4

Recall from Chapter 3 that lead aVL lies in between leads I and III with one end pointing toward the patient's left arm. This places its position at 30 and 150 degrees. Lead aVR lies in between leads I and II, placing its position also at 30 and 150 degrees, but in opposite quadrants, as one end must point toward the patient's right arm (Figure 6.5).

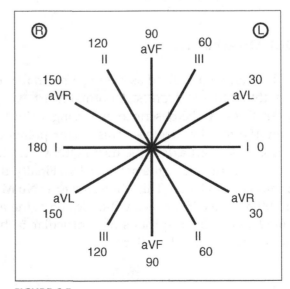

FIGURE 6.5

DEPOLARIZATION VECTORS

Each of these leads represents a distinct depolarization vector within the heart. Lead I is the separation between the negative and positive orientations above and below it. Everything below lead I has a positive orientation, because the impulses that originate here spread upward. Everything above lead I has a negative orientation, because these impulses travel downward (Figure 6.6).

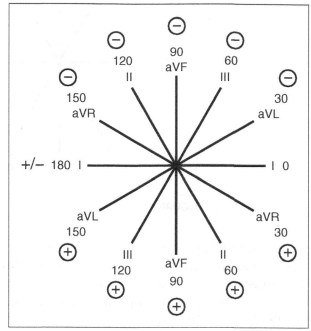

FIGURE 6.6

DEFINING THE FOUR QUADRANTS

An EKG can be described as having a **normal axis** (NML) if the mean QRS vector lies within 0 to +90 degrees. A normal heart axis points down and to the patient's left. An EKG can be described as having a **right axis** if the mean QRS vector lies within +90 to +180 degrees. This vector points down and to the patient's right. An EKG has a **left axis** if the mean QRS vector lies within 0 to −90 degrees. This vector points up and to the patient's left. Finally, the remaining quadrant depicts an extreme axis deviation. This is referred to as **No Man's Land** and falls between −180 and −90 degrees. If the mean QRS lies here, the axis is indeterminate (Figure 6.7). *Clinical Point*: Be suspicious of ventricular tachycardia or lead misplacement if there is extreme axis deviation.

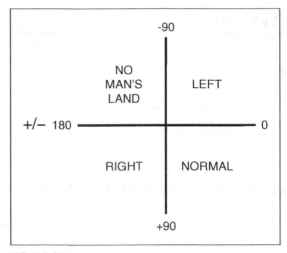

FIGURE 6.7

DETERMINING THE AXIS

Most books will discuss a complicated method for determining the axis. It is best to keep this step simple. The axis quadrant can be determined by examining **leads I and aVF**. Recall that lead I is positive on the left and negative on the right, and lead aVF is positive at the feet and negative at the head. It is where these leads overlap that defines the axis as right, left, or normal. Use Figure 6.8 for reference.

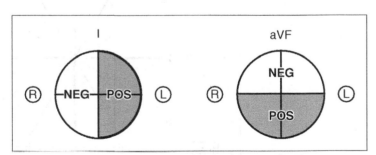

FIGURE 6.8

Begin with lead I. If the QRS is mostly positive, the axis points toward the patient's left. Next, examine lead aVF. If the QRS is negative, the axis falls in the upper left quadrant, consistent with left axis deviation (LAD). If lead I is positive and aVF is positive, the axis falls in the lower left quadrant, making the axis normal. If lead I is negative, the mean axis points to the patient's right. Now look at aVF. If the QRS is positive, the axis falls in the lower right quadrant, consistent with right axis deviation (RAD). If the QRS is negative in leads I and aVF, the axis is indeterminate. (Table 6.1)

TABLE 6.1 Axis Determination

	QRS Lead I	QRS Lead aVF
NML	Positive	Positive
LAD	Positive	Negative
RAD	Negative	Positive

SUMMARY OF AXIS QUADRANT DETERMINATION (FIGURE 6.9)

If the QRS deflection is positive in both leads I and aVF, the axis is normal. If it is positive in I and negative in aVF, there is LAD. If it is negative in I and positive in aVF, there is RAD. With these points in mind, the general axis of any EKG can be determined in seconds. This can be taken a step further to determine axis in degrees.

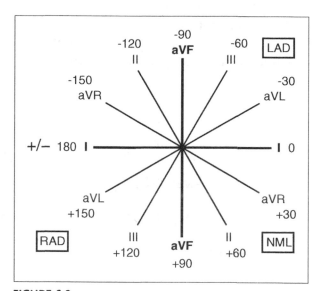

FIGURE 6.9

DETERMINING AXIS IN DEGREES

Use leads I and aVF to determine which quadrant the axis falls into: normal, left, or right. (Table 6.2) Identify the lead on EKG that is as much positive as it is negative, or isoelectric. The mean QRS vector will intersect the most isoelectric lead at a 90-degree angle. Using Figure 6.10, locate the position of this lead in the lower two quadrants. From there, move 90 degrees in the direction of the positive QRS, moving toward the quadrant already determined based on the leads I and aVF. The approximate axis can be determined in degrees using 0, 30, 60, 90, 120, 150, and 180 degrees, which are marked. EKG 6.1 will serve as an example of this method.

Step 1: Which quadrant does the axis fall in?

Lead I: positive, lead aVF: negative = LAD

Step 2: Which lead is the most isoelectric?

Lead II: +60 degrees

Step 3: From the most isoelectric lead, move 90 degrees toward the quadrant determined in Step 1.

−30 degrees

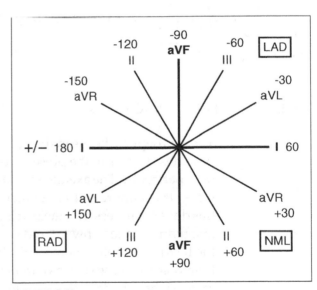

FIGURE 6.10

TABLE 6.2

	I	aVF
NML	+	+
LAD	+	−
RAD	−	+

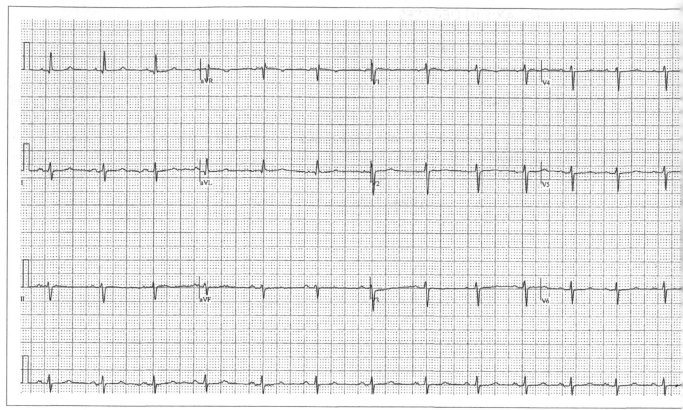

EKG 6.1

APPLYING AXIS TO CLINICAL PRACTICE

The axis depicts the mean direction of energy flow through the heart. Importantly, it provides clues as to the presence of myocardial injury, such as ischemia, infarction, or hypertrophy. The axis also can also reflect conduction system disease such as heart block. It is important to note that if the axis does not fall in the normal quadrant, this does not necessarily mean it is abnormal. If someone is obese, increased abdominal tissue pushes upward and can cause a more leftward axis. In tall, thin people, the heart can stretch more vertically, resulting in right axis deviation (Figure 6.11). Pulmonary disease such as chronic obstructive pulmonary disease (COPD) can also cause right axis deviation due to hyperinflation of the lungs, which stretches the mediastinum in a vertical direction.

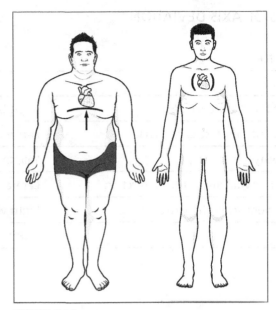

FIGURE 6.11

Additional electrical forces are needed to depolarize thickened myocardium present in ventricular hypertrophy. This results in axis deviation toward the side of the hypertrophy. If a patient has had a myocardial infarction, the area of scar tissue does not depolarize. There are no electrical vectors present. Therefore, the mean axis will point away from the area of infarction (Figure 6.12). Further clinical significance of right and left axis deviation will be reviewed with regard to bundle branch blocks, ischemia, and infarction in Chapters 7 and 8.

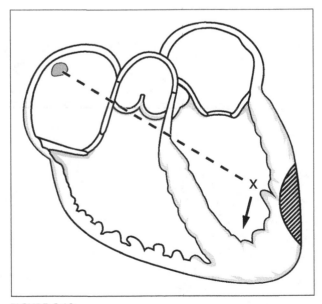

FIGURE 6.12

COMMON CAUSES OF AXIS DEVIATION

TABLE 6.3

LAD	RAD
Left bundle branch block	Right bundle branch block
Left anterior fascicular block	Left posterior fascicular block
Obesity	Tall, thin frame
Inferior wall myocardial infarction	Lateral wall myocardial infarction
Left ventricular hypertrophy	Right ventricular hypertrophy
	COPD

CHAPTER 6 REVIEW QUESTIONS

1. Determine the axis present in each of these EKGs:

   EKG 6.2

   EKG 6.3

   EKG 6.4

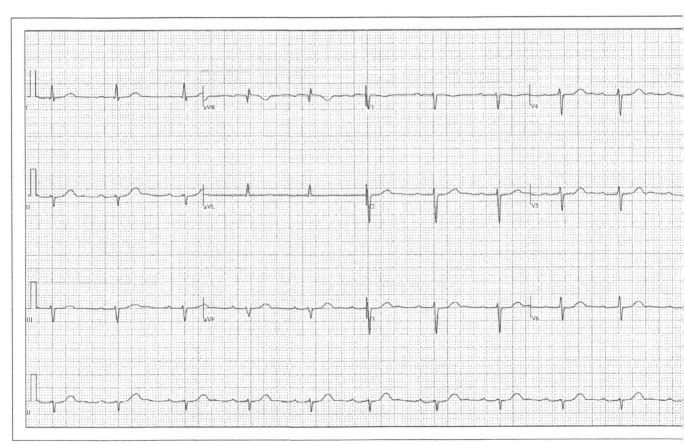

EKG 6.2

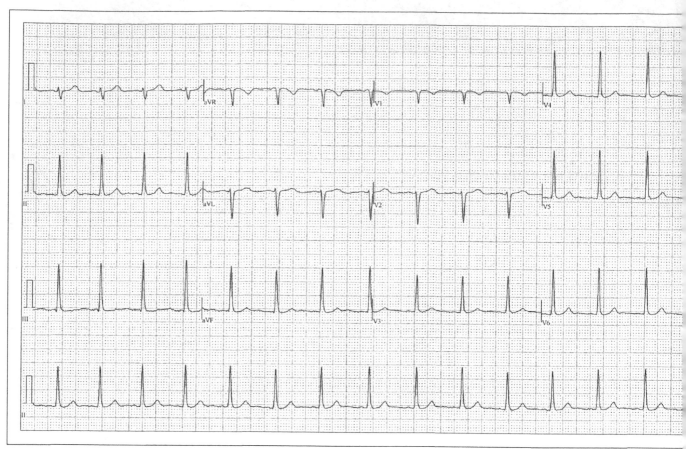

EKG 6.3

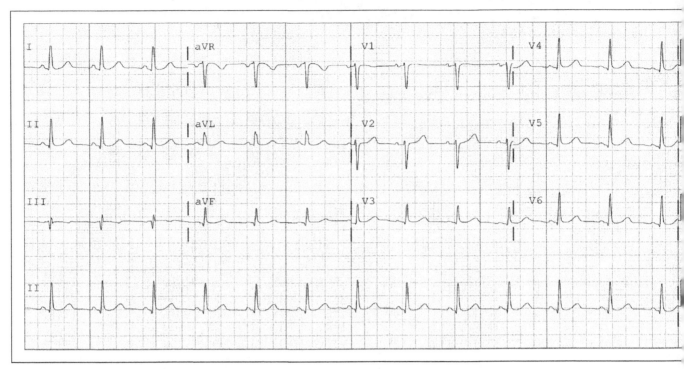

EKG 6.4

Heart Block

INTRODUCTION

Heart block is defined by the exact location of conduction delay. Heart block can occur at the level of the **sinus node**, the **atrioventricular (AV) node**, or within the **bundle branches**. Normal sinus activity starts in the sinus node and is seen on the EKG as a P wave. The conduction spreads through the atria to the AV node. This is seen as the PR interval on the EKG. The bundle of His is located just distal to the AV node and is not independently reflected by a particular interval on the EKG. From there, the conduction splits into the right and left bundle branches as they race through the ventricles. This is seen on the EKG as the QRS complex. These are the main areas to examine in the diagnosis of heart block.

SINUS PAUSE

Sinus pause, or sinus arrest, occurs when the normal sinus node fails to pace for at least one cycle before resuming normal function. The diagnosis is made by identifying the loss of a P wave. The next cycle may return with a P wave, or if the sinus node pauses long enough, there may be a junctional escape focus that temporarily takes over.

All the P waves will still have the same morphology because the atrial impulse does not change but rather temporarily blocks (EKG 7.1). This is a form of sick sinus syndrome. Such patients are prone to resting bradycardia, prolonged pauses, and chronotropic incompetence. They can also have tachycardia–bradycardia syndrome, which is associated with rapid supraventricular tachycardia alternating with profound bradycardia. Heart rate–slowing medications can exacerbate underlying sick sinus syndrome. *Clinical Point*: Sinus slowing and sinus arrest may occur during sleep. This can be associated with obstructive sleep apnea.

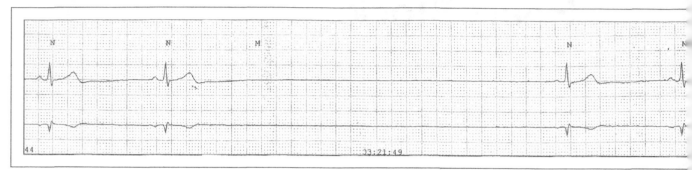

EKG 7.1

ATRIOVENTRICULAR BLOCK

AV block occurs when there is a delay or block in the impulse as it spreads from the atria to the ventricles. A block in the impulse results in a dropped QRS complex. Frequently, it is the result of a calcified and worn-down conduction system that occurs with aging; however, other precipitating causes should be ruled out. Ischemic heart disease can cause AV block, specifically if the right coronary artery is involved, as it supplies the AV node. Various rate-slowing medications can cause AV block, including calcium channel blockers, beta blockers, digoxin, and antiarrhythmic medications. Electrolyte abnormalities can cause dangerous fluctuations in electrical conduction. The most frequent culprit is potassium.

AV block can be a complication of cardiac surgery, depending on the proximity of the operating site to the conduction system. This may be temporary if it is due to procedural edema or it may be permanent if the conduction system is physically altered. Depending on the ventricular rate, AV block can cause a myriad of symptoms. These can range from mild dizziness and fatigue to syncope with resultant bodily injury.

Defining AV Block

There are four types of **AV block**: first degree, second-degree type I, second-degree type II, and third degree or complete heart block. The type of AV block is defined by its anatomic location.

First-Degree AV Block

First-degree AV block is defined by a delay in the spread of an impulse from the sinus node to the AV node (Figure 7.1). On EKG, this is seen as a prolongation of the PR interval greater than 200 milliseconds (0.2 seconds) or one large square on EKG. There is not an actual blocking of the impulse, but rather a consistent delay as it spreads from the sinus node to the ventricles. This is the mildest form of heart block and is generally asymptomatic. It commonly occurs as a result of an aging conduction system. It can also be due to a reversible cause such as rate-slowing medications or ischemia.

First-degree AV block should be monitored with documentation of the PR interval on EKG at subsequent visits if symptoms arise or if rate-slowing medications are used, as these can prolong the PR interval. As mentioned earlier, these include anti-arrhythmic medications, digoxin, calcium channel blockers, and beta blockers. Lone first-degree AV block will have no direct bearing on ventricular conduction; therefore, the QRS duration is normal unless there is an additional type of heart block present. In EKG 7.2, notice that the interval from the start of the P wave to the R wave is greater than one large box.

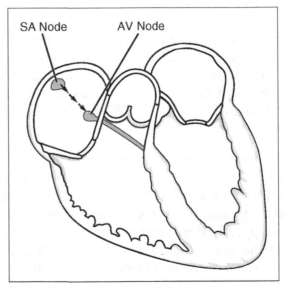

FIGURE 7.1

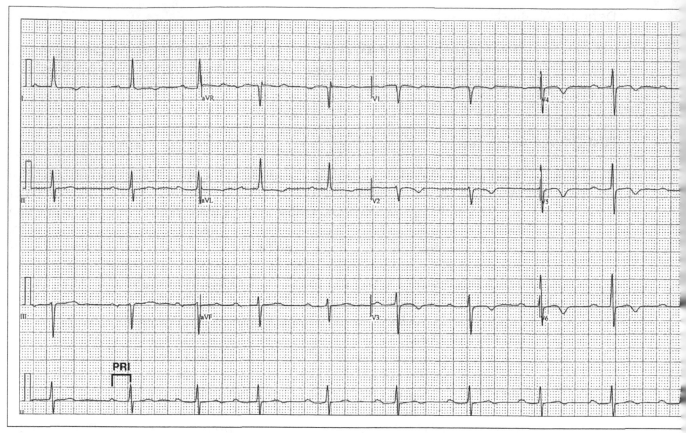

EKG 7.2

Second-Degree AV Block

There are two different types of **second-degree AV block**: Mobitz type I, also referred to as Wenckebach, and Mobitz type II. It is vital to be able to properly identify and discriminate between these two types of heart block, as one is more severe than the other. There are important distinguishing characteristics of each, which can be determined based on the anatomic location of the block.

Mobitz Type I Second-Degree AV Block (Wenckebach)

Mobitz type I is defined by a progressively lengthening PR interval from cycle to cycle prior to a dropped QRS complex. The dropped beat occurs when the AV node is no longer able to conduct a stimulus from above. The very next PR interval after the dropped beat will be significantly shorter than the PR interval of the beat just before the nonconducted P wave (EKG 7.3). Imagine someone talking to you while walking farther and farther away. Eventually, you will not be able to hear what they

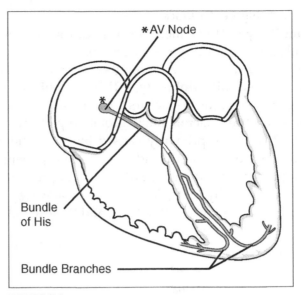

*AV Node

Bundle
of His

Bundle Branches

FIGURE 7.2

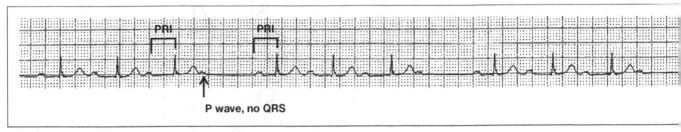

P wave, no QRS

EKG 7.3

are saying. As the impulse becomes more and more delayed, the AV node eventually and temporarily is no longer able to carry the electrical message from the sinus node.

This type of AV block is located within the AV node, and therefore, the QRS duration, reflective of conduction through the ventricles, will usually be normal (Figure 7.2). It is imperative to look at several cycles before and after each dropped beat. Be very careful to identify the dropped beat followed by a shortened PR interval.

Mobitz type I is generally asymptomatic unless there is a very slow ventricular response or if the dropped QRS is associated with a long pause. It may be reversible if associated with rate-slowing medications. Obstructive sleep apnea can also be associated with Mobitz type I heart block during sleep. This usually resolves with resolution of the apneic episodes. The treatment is aimed at removing the offending agent. If occurring in otherwise healthy individuals, it is usually temporary and intermittent. No specific treatment is indicated in asymptomatic patients. Mobitz Type I block can sometimes progress to more severe forms of AV block and if persistent, warrants monitoring.

Mobitz Type II Second-Degree AV Block

Mobitz type II is a more serious but less common type of heart block associated with a punctual P wave that is not followed by a QRS complex (EKG 7.4). The PR interval will not vary throughout cardiac cycles and, therefore, the dropped beat is unpredictable. **Mobitz type II is infra-hisian**, originating distal to the AV node (Figure 7.3). Because it occurs lower in the conduction system, the QRS will usually be wide. These factors make Mobitz type II more unstable. In contrast to Mobitz type I, it is not primarily caused by medications and is frequently irreversible. A pacemaker is typically indicated in these patients as there is a high probability for progression to complete heart block and prolonged asystole. This puts the patient at risk for bodily injury. There are several ways to differentiate Mobitz type I from Mobitz type II on a surface EKG, and these are illustrated in Table 7.1.

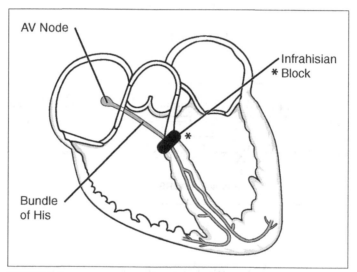

FIGURE 7.3

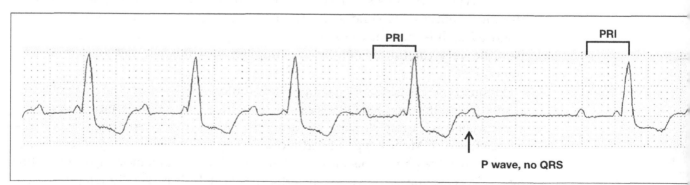

EKG 7.4

TABLE 7.1

	PR Interval	QRS Duration
Mobitz I	Gradually lengthens	Normal
Mobitz II	Fixed	Wider than normal

Distinguishing Between AV Block and Blocked PACs

Do not confuse a blocked premature atrial contraction with Mobitz type II AV block. When a dropped QRS is identified, calipers should be used to measure the atrial cycle length from P wave to P wave throughout the EKG tracing. The P wave from a blocked PAC will come in slightly early. It will depolarize the sinus node, but not the AV node. This results in a premature P wave that is not followed by a QRS. When the next P wave comes through, it results in a resetting of the overall atrial cycle length, thus creating a brief pause that can mimic a more serious form of heart block (EKG 7.5).

In contrast, Mobitz type II is defined by punctual P waves unwavering in their cycle length with intermittently dropped QRS complexes. If the atrial cycle length is properly measured throughout the EKG tracing, it should be easy to differentiate between a benign blocked PAC and a much more serious Mobitz type II block.

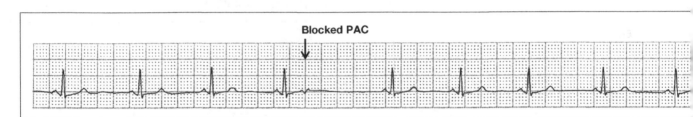

Blocked PAC

EKG 7.5

2:1 AV Block

2:1 AV block is an additional form of second-degree AV block also referred to as high-grade AV block. In 2:1 AV block, every other QRS complex is dropped. For every two atrial impulses, there is only one ventricular impulse. Because you cannot track out the P waves to see whether there is a lengthening in the PR interval, distinguishing between Mobitz type I and Mobitz type II AV block can be very difficult. If the QRS complex is wide, it is likely to be type II. If it is narrow, it is more likely to be type I. Distinguishing between the two becomes somewhat unnecessary, as any type of 2:1 AV block is generally referred to as high-grade heart block (EKG 7.6).

If symptomatic or hemodynamically unstable, temporary pacing may be recommended. If there is no reversible cause, permanent pacing is generally indicated.

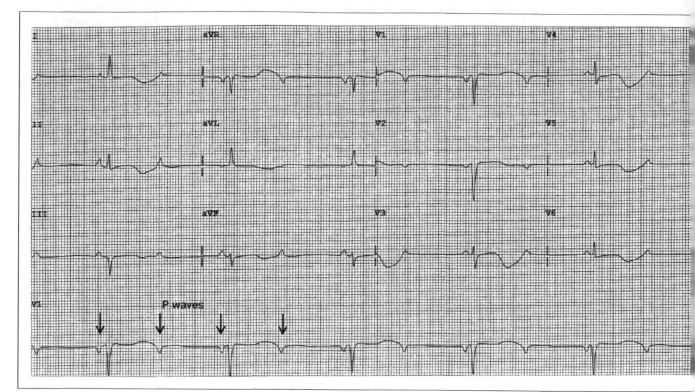

EKG 7.6

Third-Degree AV Block

Also referred to as complete heart block, **third-degree AV block** is defined by atrioventricular dissociation. None of the atrial depolarizations are able to penetrate the AV node and cause ventricular contraction. As a result, a junctional escape rhythm takes over. There are several classic findings to look for in the diagnosis of third-degree AV block. If an EKG looks suspicious for complete heart block, keep the following key points in mind:

- The ventricular rhythm is (generally) regular.

- The atrial rhythm is regular.

- There is no association between the atrial and ventricular rhythm.

- P waves are present, which could not physiologically lead to ventricular contraction.

- The atrial rate is usually normal, between 60 and 100 bpm, unless there is some form of sick sinus syndrome present as well.

- The ventricular rate is always slower than the atrial rate (EKG 7.7).

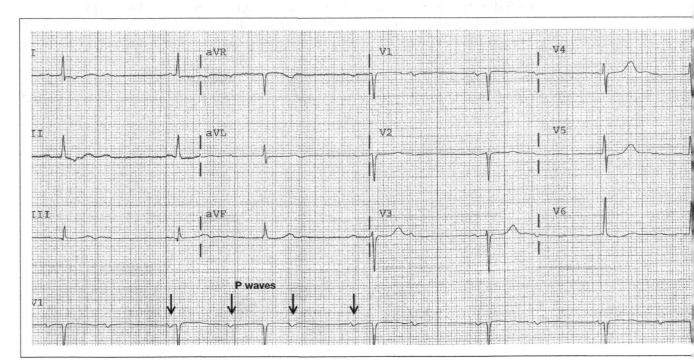

EKG 7.7

In diagnosing complete heart block, identify the location of the escape focus. Review Chapter 4. The wider and slower the QRS complex, the lower in the conduction system it originates and the more unstable it is. Complete heart block can be seen in the setting of acute myocardial infarction depending on the distribution area of the offending artery. Always interpret an EKG in its entirety. It can be easy to overlook atrioventricular dissociation in the presence of ischemic changes.

Patients with complete heart block require urgent care, especially if they are symptomatic. This indicates that their cardiac output may be severely compromised. They can be at risk for death from asystole and bodily injury from syncope. In symptomatic or unstable patients, temporary or permanent pacing is indicated, depending on the clinical scenario. If hemodynamics are compromised, agents such as atropine, dopamine, and epinephrine may be considered.

RIGHT BUNDLE AND LEFT BUNDLE BRANCH BLOCK

Ventricular conduction delay occurs when the process of ventricular depolarization takes longer than 100 milliseconds (0.1 seconds). If the QRS complex is wider than two to three small boxes on EKG paper, there is some degree of interventricular conduction delay present. Hemiblocks, or incomplete blocks, generally result in a QRS duration of 100 to 120 milliseconds (0.1–0.12 seconds), and a complete bundle branch block results in a QRS duration greater than 120 milliseconds (0.12 seconds).

Each type of block has a characteristic appearance. It is important to learn the pathophysiology involved in each type of bundle branch block to understand why the EKG appears the way it does. This will aid in understanding and not memorizing. In determining the correct diagnosis, examine the far right chest lead V1 and the far left chest lead V6 (Figure 7.4).

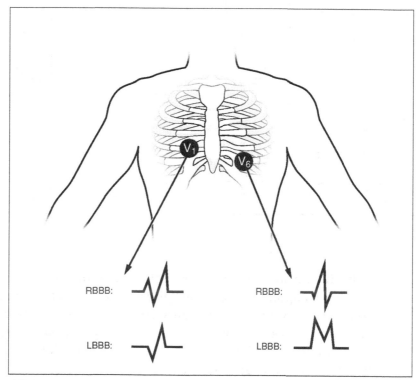

FIGURE 7.4

Normally, the electrical conduction spreads through the AV node, splits into a right and left bundle, and races down each ventricle causing them to contract almost simultaneously (Figure 7.5). If there is a delay in one bundle, conduction will slowly spread through the surrounding myocardium around the block. The unblocked bundle branch will contract sooner and depolarize the surrounding myocardium all the way across the septum, causing passive depolarization of the other ventricle. This mechanism results in a wide appearing QRS complex.

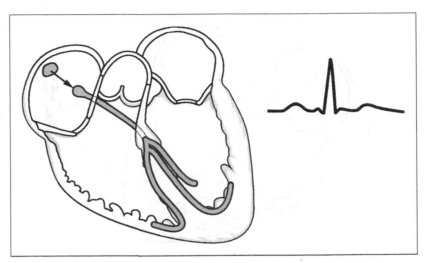

FIGURE 7.5

The more extensive the conduction block, the wider the QRS will be. If there is simply a delay in the conduction through one bundle branch, passive depolarization will begin to occur via the unblocked bundle branch, and active depolarization will catch up in the affected bundle branch. When there is a complete block in the conduction through one bundle branch, the QRS is very wide. This reflects the length of time it takes for passive depolarization to make its way across the septum. The morphologies that characteristically comprise each bundle branch block occur as a result of the mechanism and the direction of ventricular depolarization, that is, active or passive and left or right.

Right Bundle Branch Block

Right bundle branch block (RBBB) has a classic "bunny ear" appearance in the right chest leads. This is because the left ventricle contracts before the right ventricle, resulting in two joined but out of sync QRS complexes on the EKG (Figure 7.6). This causes an R, R' (R prime) pattern, which is most evident in leads V1 to V2, sometimes extending to lead V3. RBBB typically causes a qRS or RS complex with a broad S wave in lead V6 (EKG 7.8).

These typical EKG findings are due to slow, rightward spread of ventricular depolarization from the left ventricle:

- In leads V1 and V2, the R wave represents left ventricular activation and R' represents right ventricular activation occurring slightly later.

- In lead V6, the tall R wave represents left ventricular activation occurring first and an S wave represents right ventricular activation occurring slightly later via the left ventricle.

- Right axis deviation is frequently seen in the setting of a RBBB.

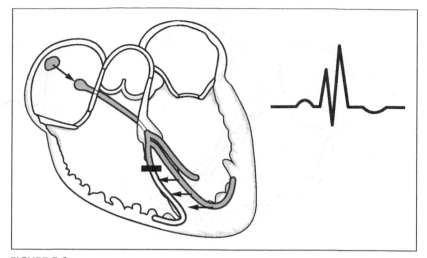

FIGURE 7.6

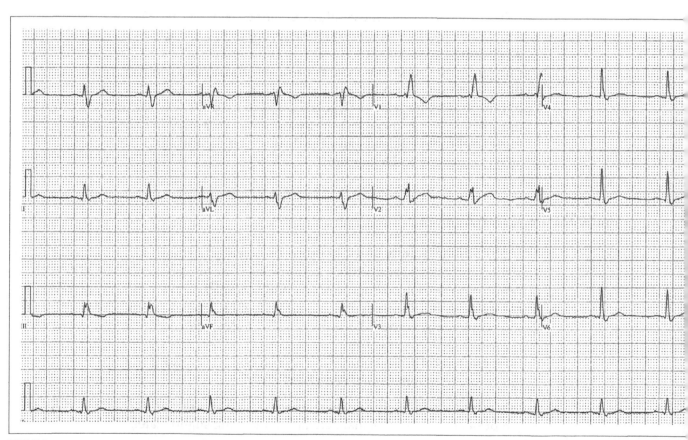

EKG 7.8

Causes of RBBB

The presence of a RBBB is not necessarily abnormal. It can occur in structurally normal hearts and should be correlated clinically. It can occur as a result of normal aging in patients with fibrocalcific conduction disease. It can be abnormal, occurring in any condition that affects the right side of the heart. This includes atrial septal defect, right ventricular hypertrophy, pulmonary stenosis, pulmonary arterial hypertension, or pulmonary embolus.

If a RBBB is present, consider the clinical presentation. This will help determine whether further action is warranted. Although isolated RBBB can be normal, concomitant heart block such as first-degree AV block or a left hemiblock should always be monitored closely. When additional areas of conduction block are present, there is a higher probability of progression to complete heart block. This may be particularly exacerbated by rate-slowing medical therapy.

Clinical Point: The right bundle branch is supplied directly by perforating branches of the left anterior descending artery. A new RBBB should not be overlooked in a patient with suspected myocardial infarction, particularly if the anterior wall is affected. This can lead to high-grade AV block and carries a poor prognosis.

Left Bundle Branch Block

Left bundle branch block (LBBB) causes the same type of widened QRS complex but has a completely different appearance from a RBBB on EKG. If a LBBB is present, the right ventricle will depolarize first and electrical activation will spread slowly over to the left ventricle (Figure 7.7).

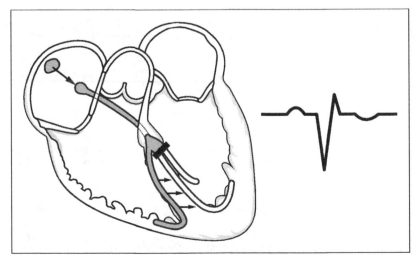

FIGURE 7.7

The classic changes seen on the EKG in a LBBB are best seen in leads V1 and V6, just like in a RBBB. Lead V1 will have a QS complex and lead V6 will have a tall R wave, frequently with R, R′ pattern and no q wave. Inverted T waves may also be seen in a LBBB (EKG 7.9).

These typical EKG findings are due to slow, leftward spread of ventricular depolarization from the right ventricle:

- A delay in total time of depolarization of the left ventricle accounts for a very wide QRS complex throughout all leads.

- The QS complex in lead V1 represents the slow spread of ventricular depolarization from right to left. The Q wave represents right ventricular depolarization, and the S wave represents left ventricular depolarization.

- Loss of (or delayed) septal depolarization results in a loss of the septal q wave in lead V6. The R wave represents right ventricular activation, whereas R′ represents left ventricular activation.

- Left axis deviation may be seen in the setting of a LBBB.

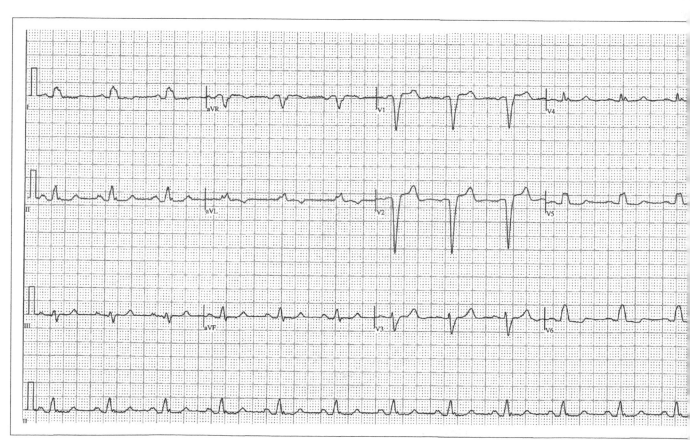

EKG 7.9

Causes of LBBB

In contrast to a RBBB, LBBB is more likely to be associated with structural heart disease. When present, LBBB creates difficulty in examining the EKG for ischemia. This is because the classic QRS and T wave changes can mimic a myocardial infarction pattern and obscure findings typically present in prior myocardial infarction. This will be reviewed in more detail in Chapter 8.

LBBB is most commonly associated with coronary artery disease or valvular heart disease, but it can also occur as a result of fibrocalcific changes. Given the size of the left bundle branch, it would require significant calcification before a conduction delay becomes evident. Always examine the EKG for additional conduction delays such as first-degree AV block or an incomplete right bundle branch block (IRBBB). Such patients are at risk for complete heart block. Always review the patient's medication list for rate-slowing medications or antiarrhythmic medications, which may potentiate the conduction disease.

Review: Diagnosing Bundle Branch Block

The first step in diagnosing a complete bundle branch block is to identify a QRS duration greater than 120 milliseconds (0.12 seconds). Second, examine leads V1 and V6 for these classic appearances to easily differentiate between RBBB and LBBB (Table 7.2).

TABLE 7.2 Diagnosing Bundle Branch Block

	V1	V6
RBBB	rSR or R, R'	qRS or RS
LBBB	QS	R wave, no Q

Right Bundle Branch Block

- R, R' in V1 to V3

- qRS or RS in V6

- Frequently right axis deviation with axis +120 or more positive

Left Bundle Branch Block

- Wide QS in V1

- Tall R wave without q wave in V6

- Frequently left axis deviation with axis −45 or more negative

RIGHT AND LEFT HEMIBLOCK

If the QRS duration is less than 120 milliseconds (0.12 seconds) but greater than 100 milliseconds (0.1 seconds), this is indicative, but not diagnostic, of a hemiblock. There are several possibilities: left anterior fascicular block (LAFB), left posterior fascicular block (LPFB), and incomplete right bundle branch block (IRBBB).

Incomplete RBBB

As previously reviewed, the left bundle branch consists of an anterior fascicle and a posterior fascicle, whereas the right bundle branch consists of a single fascicle. An IRBBB will have a similar appearance to that seen in complete right bundle branch block, but the QRS duration will be less than 120 milliseconds (0.12 seconds) (EKG 7.10). Right axis deviation is frequently present. This is a little more straightforward than left bundle hemiblock.

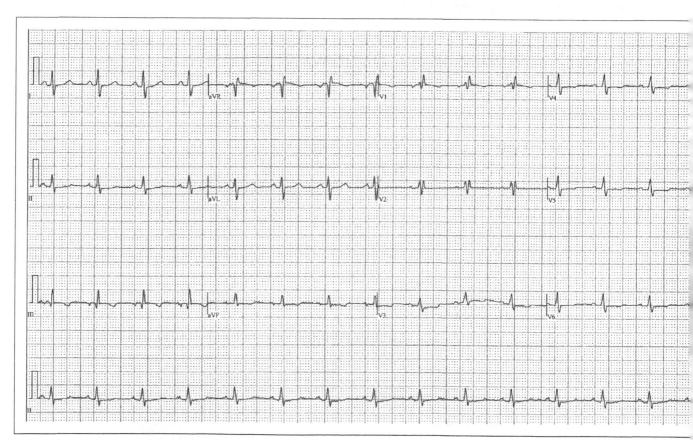

EKG 7.10

Left Bundle Hemiblock

If the QRS duration is greater than 100 milliseconds (0.1 seconds) but not quite wide enough to be diagnostic of a complete bundle branch block, then determine the axis. This is the key in distinguishing between a LAFB and LPFB. QRS duration alone does not diagnose a hemiblock as it may be normal in the setting of a hemiblock. Note the location of each fascicle, as this makes it easier to understand the EKG appearance and axis deviation associated with each (Figure 7.8).

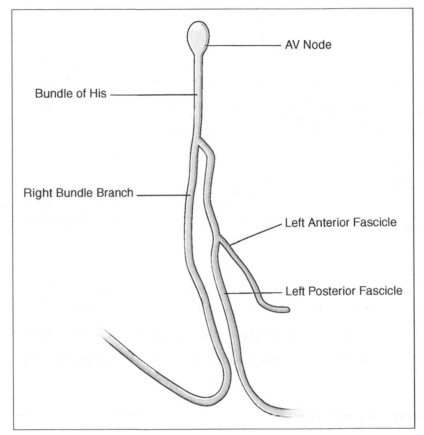

FIGURE 7.8

Left Anterior Fascicular Block

LAFB is much more common than a LPFB (EKG 7.11). The left anterior fascicle is located toward the anterolateral portion of the left ventricle. When this fascicle is blocked, there is a delay in electrical activation of this area, therefore shifting the general axis toward this direction. As a result, there is left axis deviation or an axis of −30 to −45 degrees or more negative. This delayed (but not absent) activation also

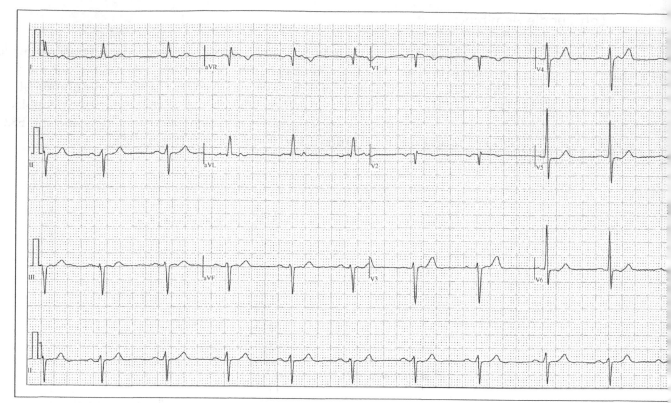

EKG 7.11

results in an RS pattern in the lateral precordial lead V6. There are two main findings on EKG that must be present to diagnose a LAFB:

- An rS pattern in the inferior leads and qR pattern in the lateral leads
- Left axis deviation with axis −30 to −45 or more negative

Left Posterior Fascicular Block

The left posterior fascicle is located more inferiorly and toward the right side of the left ventricle. When this fascicle is blocked, there is a delay in the electrical activation of this area, therefore shifting the axis toward the right. This results in right axis deviation or an axis of +120 or more positive (EKG 7.12). The EKG findings are just the opposite of that seen in LAFB and include

- qR pattern in the inferior leads and rS pattern in the lateral leads
- Right axis deviation with axis +120 or more positive

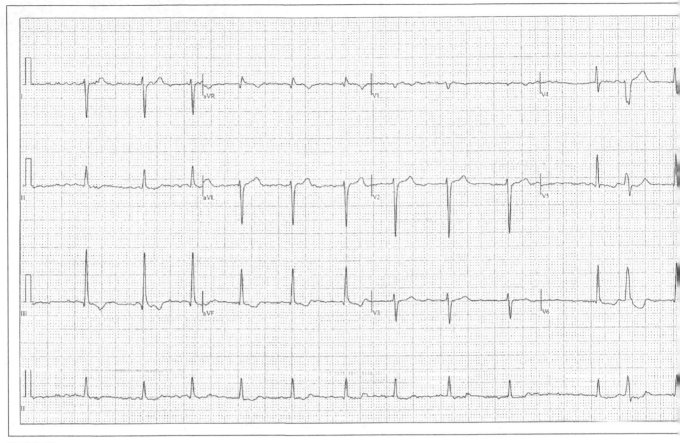

EKG 7.12

If the QRS duration is 100 to 120 milliseconds (0.1 to 0.12 seconds) and the EKG does not meet the criteria in Table 7.3, this is referred to more simply as an interventricular conduction delay.

TABLE 7.3 Diagnostic Criteria for Left Hemiblock

	Inferior Leads	Lateral Leads	Axis
LAFB	rS: QRS negative	qR: QRS positive	Left (−30 or more negative)
LPFB	qR: QRS positive	rS: QRS negative	Right (+120 or more positive)

CHAPTER 7 REVIEW QUESTIONS

1. An interventricular conduction delay is defined by a QRS duration > _____ milliseconds.

2. A gradually lengthening PRi followed by a dropped QRS and a subsequent shorter PRi is diagnostic of _____ heart block.

3. Define the type of conduction delay present in each of these EKGs.

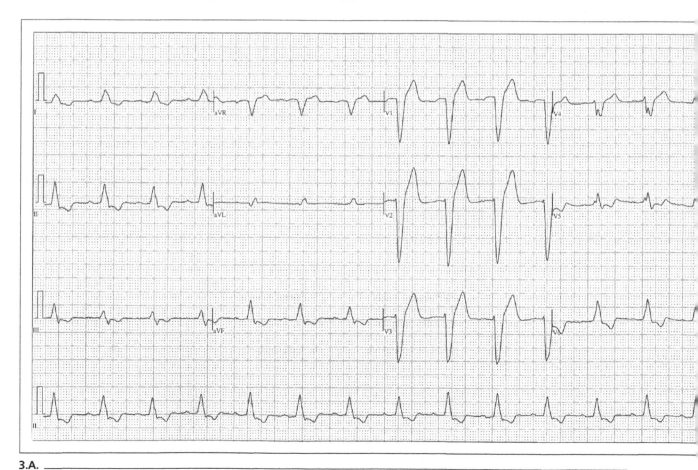

3.A. _____

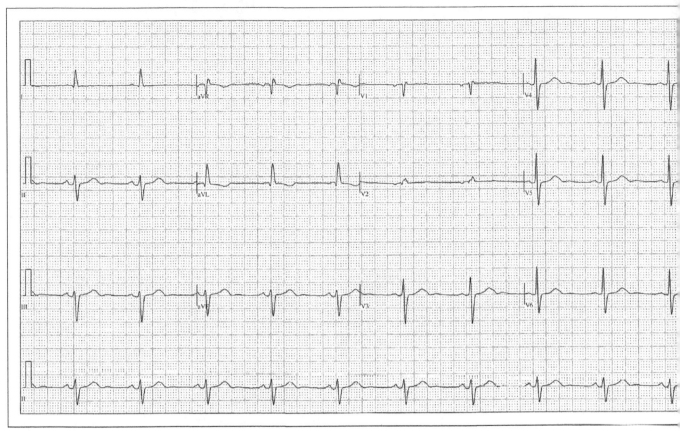

3.B.

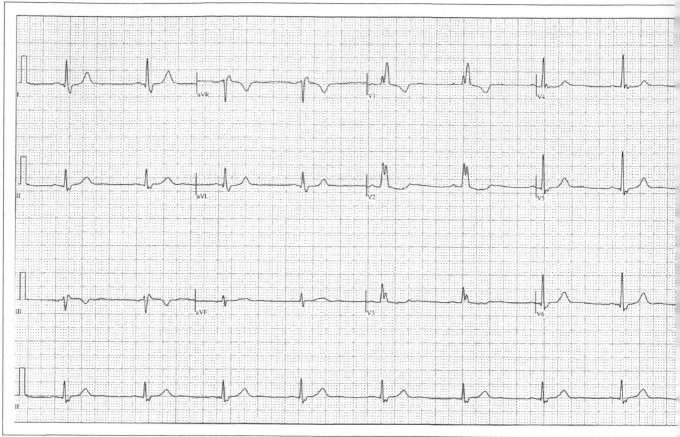

3.C. _____

4. Dissociation of regular P waves from regular QRS complexes defines _____ heart block.

5. LAFB causes _____ axis deviation.

6. LPFB causes _____ axis deviation.

7. Which type of second-degree heart block carries more immediate concern?

Ischemia and Infarction

INTRODUCTION

Ischemia occurs when there is a narrowing in one of the coronary arteries resulting in decreased blood flow and tissue hypoxemia. Diminished blood flow causes a change in the depolarization and repolarization pattern; that is, it is delayed but not absent. If the ischemia extends through the entire thickness of the ventricular wall, infarction is imminent.

Infarction occurs when there is a complete obstruction of one of the coronary arteries that supplies a particular area of the myocardium. This results in tissue death and a lack of depolarization. This changes the way electricity flows through the affected area of the heart, causing specific patterns we can look for on EKG to aid in the diagnosis.

ISCHEMIA

Ischemia occurs in several stages, depicted in Figure 8.1. Ischemia is initially represented by T wave inversion (EKG 8.1). This is the first clue that there is some degree of obstructed blood flow. The affected T wave should be symmetrically inverted. One side should not be more inverted than the other.

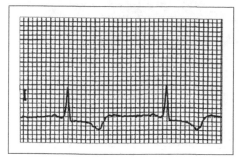

EKG 8.1

When ischemia progresses through the layers of the myocardium, the EKG changes progress as well. ST segment depression occurs when ischemia has extended further into the deeper layers of the myocardium (EKG 8.2). This is an unstable finding that is reflective of increased myocardial demand due to worsening ischemia. ST depression is a warning sign that infarction may soon occur.

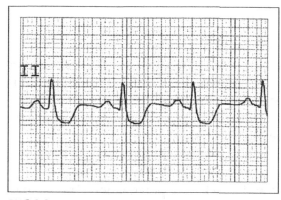

EKG 8.2

ST segment elevation is reflective of the early stages of infarction and is referred to as an injury pattern (EKG 8.3). ST segment elevation and depression should be defined in millimeters from baseline. In general, anything ≥2 mm, or 2 small boxes, is clinically significant. At this point, the process of infarction is ongoing or imminent, and these findings should be treated as such.

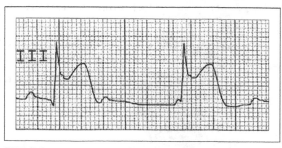

EKG 8.3

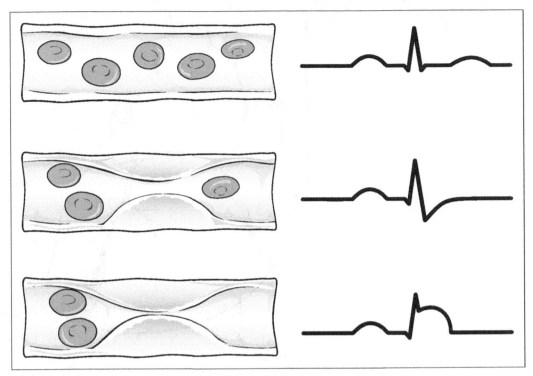

FIGURE 8.1

INFARCTION

Infarction is represented by a Q wave or the first downward deflection after the P wave (EKG 8.4). Q waves occur because there is an alteration of blood flow at the cellular level. Scar tissue does not properly depolarize or repolarize, and therefore, electricity essentially reroutes around the affected area (Figure 8.2). Deep Q waves are often associated with inverted T waves reflective of this process. Q waves ≥2 mm are indicative of previous myocardial infarction. Serial EKGs are a vital part of a chest pain workup based on the mechanisms involved in the progression of ischemia and infarction.

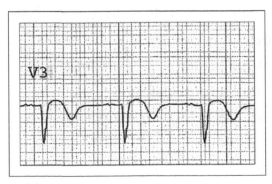

EKG 8.4

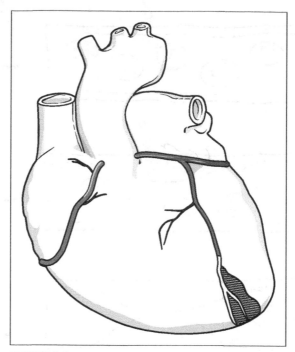

FIGURE 8.2

Scar tissue created after myocardial infarction does not depolarize, and there-fore, electrical vectors point away from areas of injury. For example, recall from Chapter 3 that leads I and aVL represent positive vectors at the left arm. If there is an obstruction in an artery that supplies the left lateral wall, such as the left circumflex artery, this part of the myocardium will no longer depolarize. Electrical vectors will point away from this area (Figure 8.3). This explains why infarction is represented by negative forces on the EKG, that is, Q waves and inverted T waves.

CORONARY BLOOD SUPPLY (FIGURE 8.4)

- The right coronary artery (RCA)

  - Right ventricle

  - Inferior portion of the left ventricle

  - Atrioventricular (AV) node

  - The conal branch of the RCA supplies the sinus node

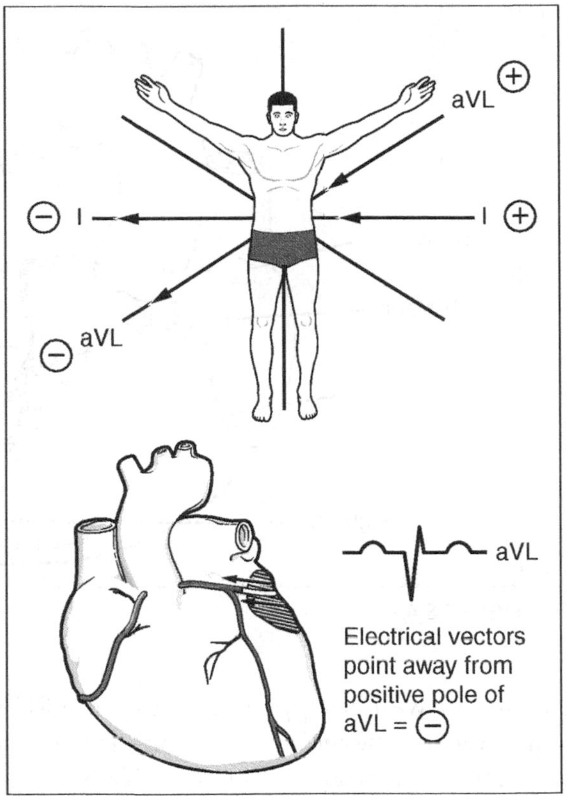

FIGURE 8.3

- The left anterior descending (LAD) artery
  - Anterior portion of the left ventricle
  - Interventricular septum
  - Perforating branches of the left anterior descending artery supply the right bundle branch and left bundle branch
- The left circumflex artery
  - Lateral wall of the left ventricle
  - Less commonly, supplies the sinus node and/or the AV node

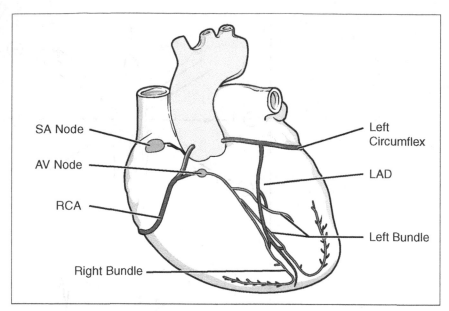

FIGURE 8.4

The posterior wall is supplied by either the RCA or the left circumflex artery. It is supplied by whichever artery is dominant in the coronary circulation and wraps around the heart to supply the majority of the posterior wall. Based on this information, ischemic changes in corresponding leads can be examined on the EKG to determine which major artery has been compromised. (Table 8.1)

TABLE 8.1 Coronary Distribution

	EKG Leads	**Myocardial Distribution**
RCA	II, III, aVF	Inferior wall
LAD	V1–V4	Anterior wall
Left circumflex	I, aVL, V5–V6	Lateral wall

CORONARY SUPPLY TO CONDUCTION SYSTEM

Based on the coronary blood supply to the conduction system, myocardial infarction can be complicated by underlying heart block (Table 8.2). When present, this generally carries a worse prognosis. These changes may be temporary if the ischemia is corrected quickly. If extensive infarction is present, the heart block may be irreversible.

- Inferior wall myocardial infarction can be associated with sinus arrest or complete heart block, as the RCA supplies the AV node and the sinus node.

- Anterior infarction can be complicated by a new bundle branch block or complete heart block, as the left anterior descending artery supplies the interventricular septum.

TABLE 8.2 Coronary Supply to Conduction System

Coronary Artery	Conduction System Supplied
Right coronary	SA node, AV node
Left anterior descending	Right bundle branch Left bundle branch
Left circumflex	SA node (less common) AV node (less common)

FOLLOWING A PATTERN

The importance of following a pattern when interpreting a 12-lead EKG is especially vital when diagnosing ischemia and infarction. Carefully examine the inferior leads, lateral leads, and anterior leads as individual groups, remembering which major coronary artery supplies which section. This will help narrow the focus to the affected area. There cannot be ischemia/infarction present if the changes are not present in contiguous leads. For example, if there is a Q wave in lead III but not in lead II and aVF, this is not diagnostic of an old inferior wall myocardial infarction. This should be interpreted as a nonspecific finding.

RECIPROCAL CHANGES

Reciprocity is another important characteristic to remember when diagnosing myocardial injury. The primary injury is represented by ST elevation, whereas the reciprocal change is represented by ST depression:

- Anterior wall injury will cause reciprocal changes in the inferior leads.

- Lateral wall injury will cause reciprocal changes in the inferior leads.

- Inferior wall injury will cause reciprocal changes in the lateral leads.

- Posterior wall injury will cause reciprocal changes in the anterior leads.

For example, in the setting of acute anterior wall injury, there will be ST segment elevation in V1–V4 and ST depression in II, III, and aVF. Look for these reciprocal changes to help confirm the diagnosis.

ANTERIOR WALL ISCHEMIA AND INFARCTION

The anterior myocardium is supplied by the left anterior descending artery (Figure 8.5). Evidence of ischemia affecting the anterior wall is seen by examining the ST segment and T waves in the precordial chest leads V1–V4. An injury pattern in these leads is almost always associated with reciprocal changes in the inferior leads II, III, and aVF. Anterior wall ischemia will cause T wave inversion in leads V1 to V4 in the early stages. As the ischemia progresses, this is reflected by ST segment depression in V1 to V4. Ongoing injury is reflected by ST segment elevation in these leads (EKG 8.5). Transmural infarction is represented by Q waves in leads V1 to V4 (EKG 8.6).

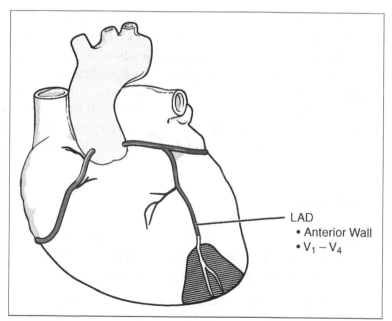

LAD
- Anterior Wall
- $V_1 - V_4$

FIGURE 8.5

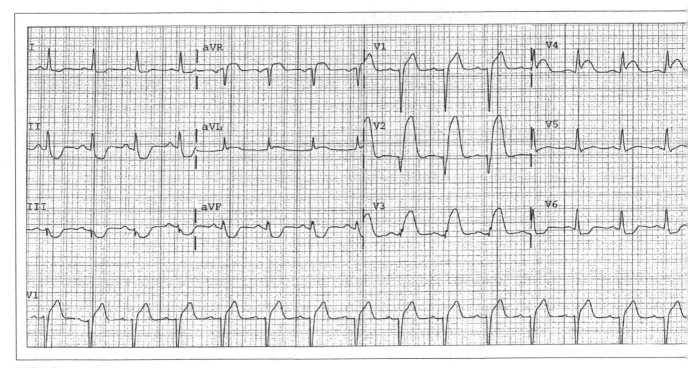

EKG 8.5

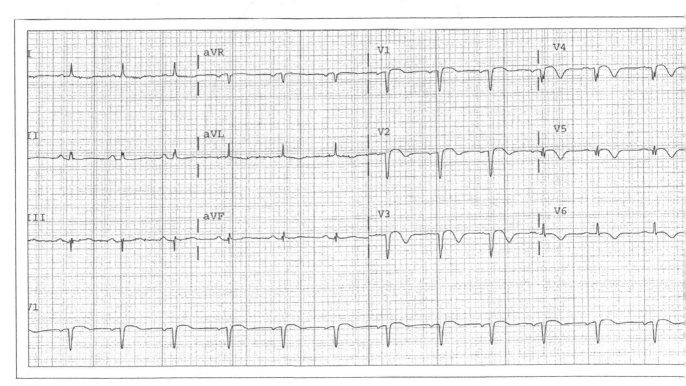

EKG 8.6

LATERAL WALL ISCHEMIA AND INFARCTION

The lateral wall is supplied by the left circumflex artery (Figure 8.6). Evidence of ischemia affecting the lateral wall is seen by examining the ST segment and T waves in leads I and aVL, and also the lateral precordial leads V5 and V6. Reciprocal changes are usually seen in leads II, III, and aVF when an injury pattern is present. Initially, lateral wall ischemia will cause T wave inversion in leads I, aVL, V5, and V6, whereas progressive ischemia is reflected by ST segment depression in these leads. Ongoing injury is seen as ST segment elevation (EKG 8.7). Transmural infarction is represented by Q waves in these leads (EKG 8.8).

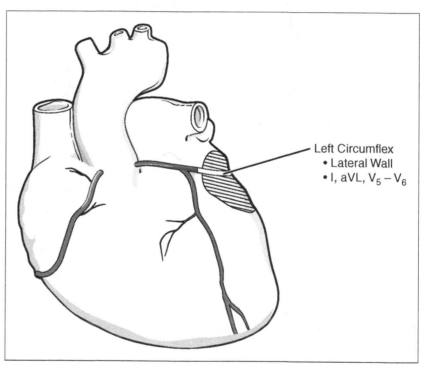

Left Circumflex
• Lateral Wall
• I, aVL, $V_5 - V_6$

FIGURE 8.6

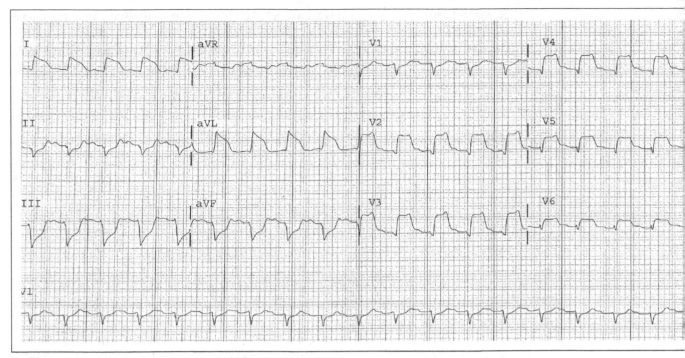

EKG 8.7

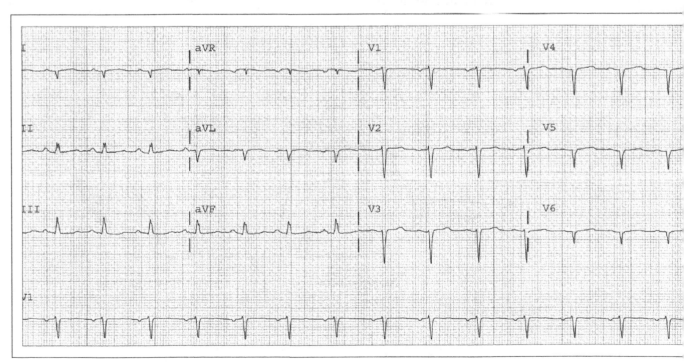

EKG 8.8

Refer to Figure 8.3. A lateral wall myocardial infarction will often cause right axis deviation because electrical vectors point away from the area of injury. Note the right axis deviation present in EKG 8.8. This is not a left posterior fascicular block, because leads I and aVL have Q waves. True LPFB will have an rS pattern in these leads, without a Q wave.

INFERIOR WALL ISCHEMIA AND INFARCTION

The inferior myocardium is supplied by the RCA (Figure 8.7). Evidence of ischemia affecting the inferior wall is seen by examining the ST segment and T waves in the inferior leads II, III, and aVF. Reciprocal changes are usually seen in leads I, aVL, and V5 to V6 when an injury pattern is present. Inferior wall ischemia will cause T wave inversions in leads II, III, and aVF. Progressive ischemia is reflected by ST depression. Ongoing injury will cause ST segment elevation (EKG 8.9). Transmural infarction is reflected by Q waves in the inferior leads (EKG 8.10). The RCA also supplies the AV node. Acute inferior wall injury is sometimes associated with complete heart block (EKG 8.11).

Inferior wall myocardial infarction will often cause left axis deviation because the electrical vectors will point away from the area of injury. Note the left axis deviation present in EKG 8.10. This is not a true left anterior fascicular block because leads II, III, and aVF have Q waves present. LAFB by definition will have an rS pattern in the inferior leads.

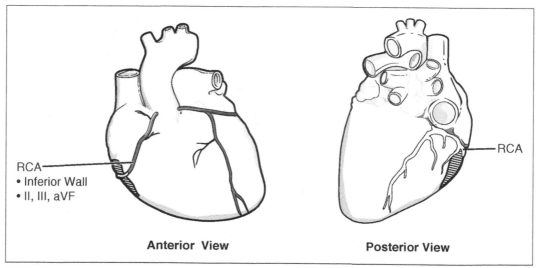

FIGURE 8.7

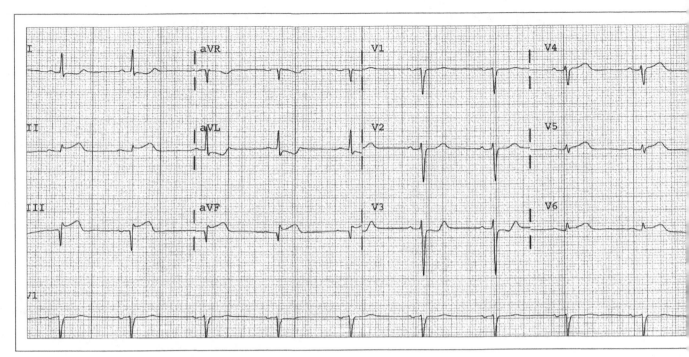

EKG 8.9

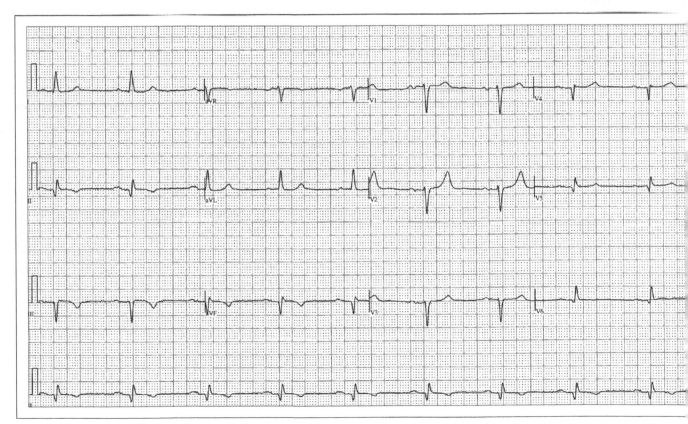

EKG 8.10

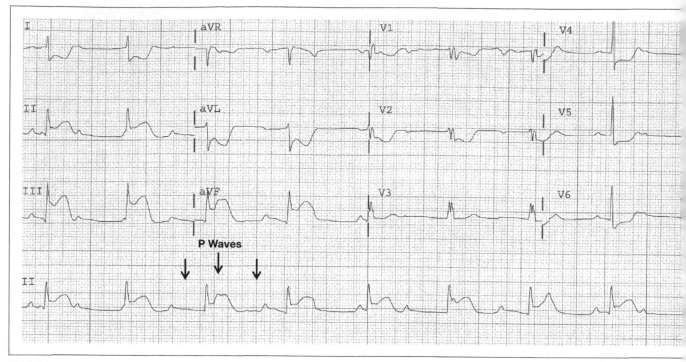

EKG 8.11

POSTERIOR WALL ISCHEMIA AND INFARCTION

Isolated posterior infarction is rarely seen. It almost always occurs in the setting of inferior or lateral wall myocardial infarction. It can be caused by an obstruction in either the RCA or the left circumflex artery, depending on which supplies the majority of the posterior wall (Figure 8.8). Posterior ischemia and infarction can be more difficult to diagnose, because the typical lead placement in a standard 12-lead EKG does not allow for a good look at the posterior wall. Therefore, we must rely on reciprocal changes seen in the anterior leads as depolarization of the anterior wall is exactly opposite to that of the posterior wall. An anterior wall myocardial infarction is diagnosed by ST segment elevation and Q waves in the precordial leads. Posterior wall ischemia produces an opposite picture, with tall R waves and deep S waves typically seen in the right chest leads along with ST segment depression (EKG 8.12). This EKG example shows evidence of concomitant acute inferior wall injury.

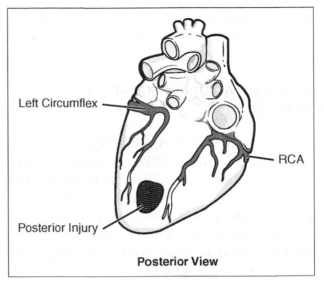

FIGURE 8.8

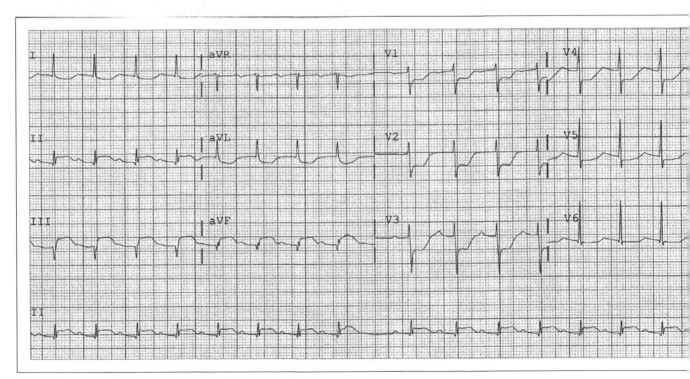

EKG 8.12

If these findings are noted, perform a "mirror test." Look at the EKG in a mirror or flip it upside down and hold it up to a light looking at the back side. If Q waves and ST elevation are seen in leads V1 to V3, there is likely a posterior myocardial infarction underway. Progression of posterior wall injury is reflected by the development of a smaller R wave and a larger S wave.

EVALUATING FOR ISCHEMIA IN THE PRESENCE OF BUNDLE BRANCH BLOCK

Right bundle branch blocks (RBBBs) do not typically obscure findings of ischemia or infarction, because a RBBB affects predominantly the end of ventricular depolarization. Ischemia, infarction, and left bundle branch block (LBBB) affect both the early and late phases of ventricular depolarization. By definition, LBBB is reflected by Q waves, ST segment, and T wave changes and the loss of normal R wave progression. These are the same findings that can be present in ischemia and infarction. Note the appearance of normal R wave progression in EKG 8.13 compared with the R wave progression in LBBB in EKG 8.14.

As detailed by Sgarbossa, Pinski, Gates, and Wagner (1996), there are specific criteria for diagnosing ischemia in the presence of a LBBB or right ventricular paced complexes, which cause a LBBB appearance. These are often referred to as Sgarbossa's criteria and include:

- ST elevation > 1 mm in leads with a positive QRS complex (QRS concordant with ST segment)

- ST depression > 1 mm in V1 to V3

- ST elevation > 5 mm in leads with a negative QRS complex (QRS discordant with ST segment)

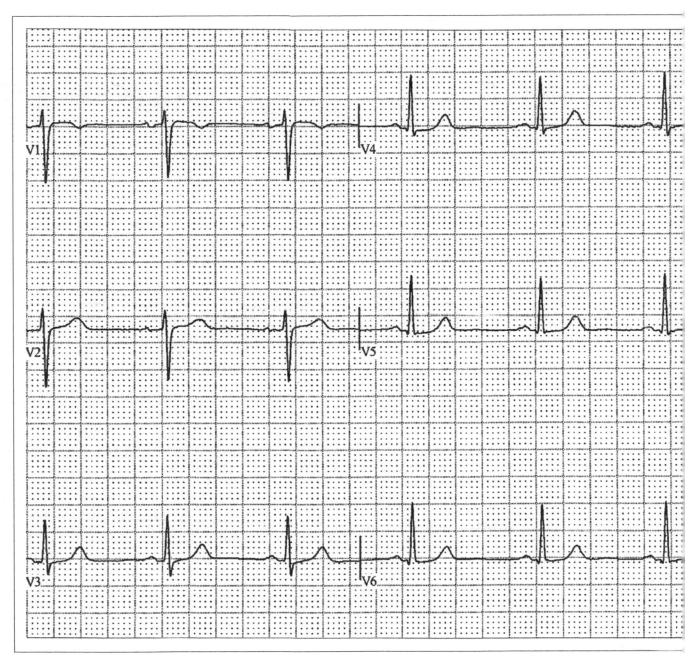

EKG 8.13

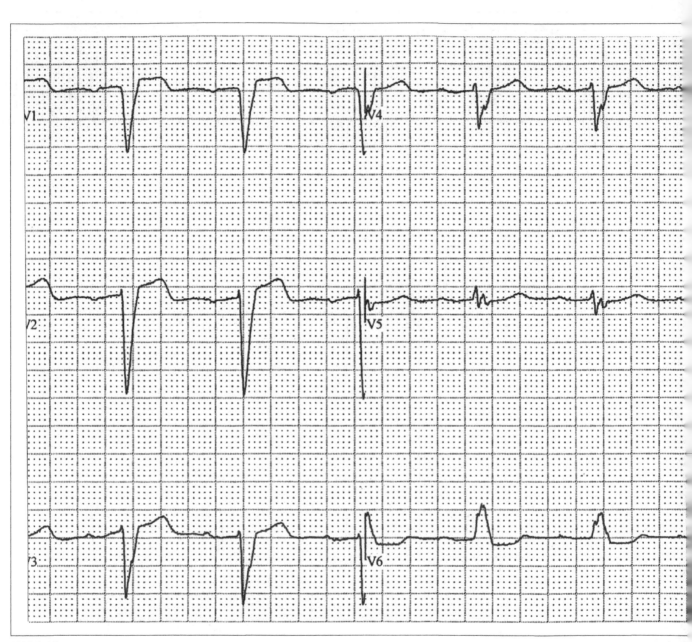

EKG 8.14

Note the significant ST elevation present in the anterior leads in EKG 8.15. In this example, the ST segment elevation is discordant with the QRS and exceeds 5 mm.

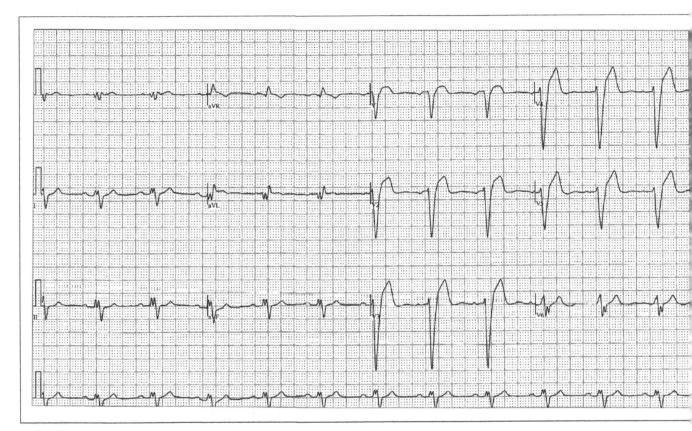

EKG 8.15

Do not overlook the importance of serial EKGs in the presence of a LBBB. ST and T wave changes will still evolve in the setting of an infarction, although they can be more subtle in the presence of an interventricular conduction delay. The patient of EKG 8.16 complained of anginal-type symptoms that improved by the time he presented to the emergency department. A repeat EKG was ordered when he began to experience crescendo anginal symptoms. Note the significant ST and T wave changes present in multiple precordial leads in EKG 8.17. This patient was in the midst of an acute anterior wall myocardial infarction and underwent emergent percutaneous intervention.

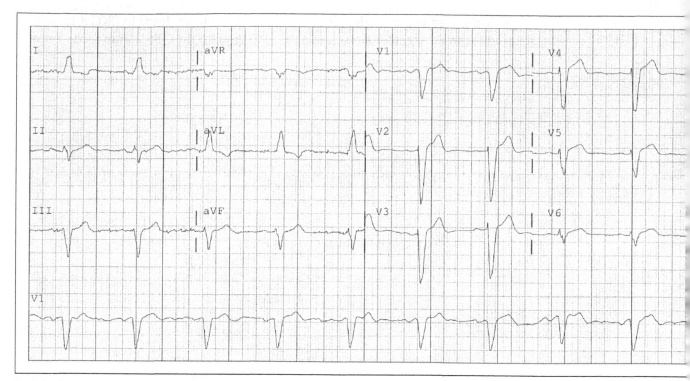

EKG 8.16

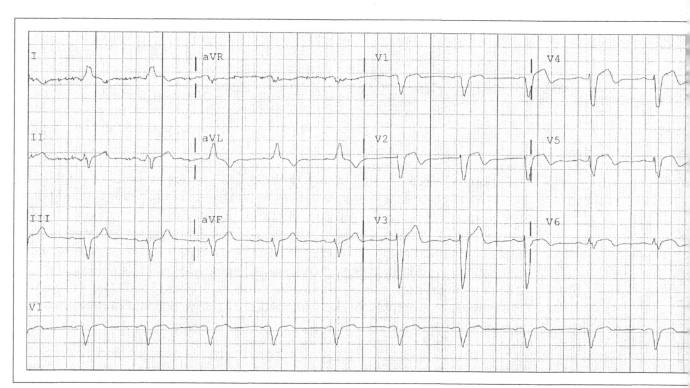

EKG 8.17

EKG FINDINGS IN VENTRICULAR ANEURYSM

Ventricular aneurysms are areas of severely weakened myocardium lined with scar tissue that can be a complication of an extensive myocardial infarction (Figure 8.9). They are more commonly associated with anterior and inferior wall myocardial infarction. This area of weakened heart muscle does not contract normally during systole. On EKG, this is seen as persistent ST elevation after MI (EKG 8.18). Unlike ST elevation in acute myocardial infarction, which resolves within days, this can persist weeks and even months after the injury. *Clinical Point*: Ventricular aneurysms are a poor prognostic finding and can be associated with ventricular arrhythmias and progression of congestive heart failure.

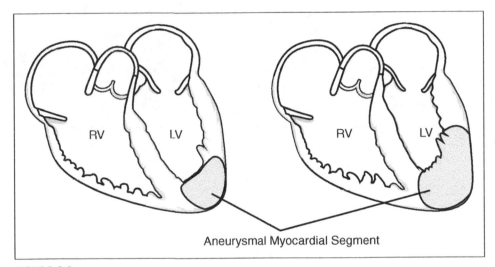

Aneurysmal Myocardial Segment

FIGURE 8.9

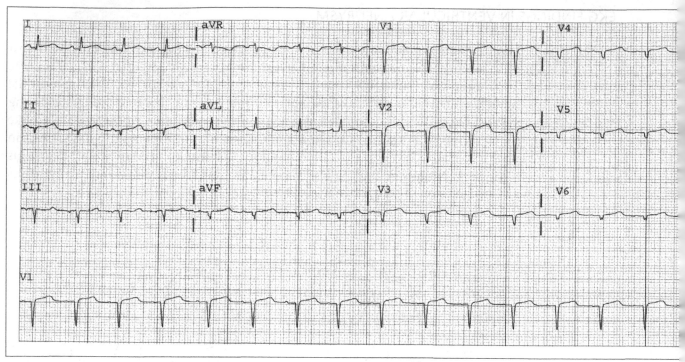

EKG 8.18

CHAPTER 8 REVIEW QUESTIONS

1. T wave inversion is indicative of _____.

2. An old myocardial infarction is represented on EKG by _____.

3. Which type of bundle branch block makes evaluating for ischemia more difficult?

4. Acute anterior wall injury will cause primary changes in leads _____ and reciprocal changes in leads _____.

5. Acute inferior wall injury will cause primary changes in leads _____ and reciprocal changes in leads _____.

6. Acute lateral wall injury will cause primary changes in leads _____ and reciprocal changes in leads _____.

7. Ventricular aneurysms cause which type of persistent pattern on EKG?

8. Which main coronary artery is the likely cause of the injury or infarct patterns seen in the following EKGs?

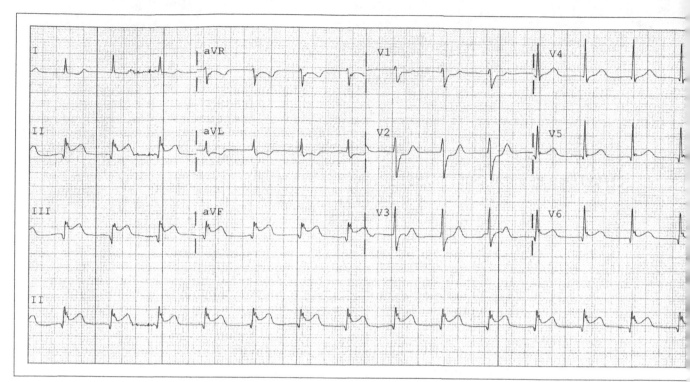

8.A. _____

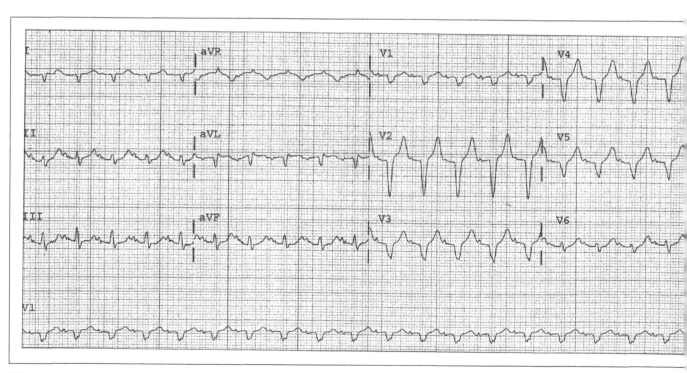

8.B. _____

Supraventricular Tachycardia

INTRODUCTION

Supraventricular tachycardia (SVT) is a common, all-encompassing term for any rapid arrhythmia that originates above the ventricles. This can include anything from sinus tachycardia to atrial fibrillation to atrioventricular (AV) node reentrant tachycardia. SVT is best understood when broken down into distinct groups. There are specific findings to look for on EKG to aid in the diagnosis. Sometimes it is not possible to determine the exact location of the SVT based on only a 12-lead EKG without an electrophysiology study. This is especially true for rhythms associated with a very rapid ventricular response. In these cases, the EKG may simply be interpreted as "SVT."

SVT causes a narrow complex QRS duration of less than 120 milliseconds (0.12 seconds), or three small boxes on an EKG. If there is aberrant or slow conduction through the ventricles, this can result in a wide-appearing QRS, which can make the diagnosis more difficult.

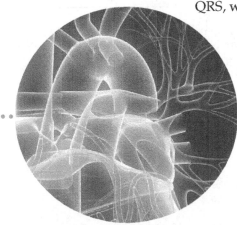

DIAGNOSING SVT

There are two main points to remember when diagnosing SVT:

1. **Identify the P wave**. The P wave may not be always visible, but when identifiable, it holds the key to the diagnosis.

   • Look for a break or a pause in the rhythm. This is a good place to pick out P waves and note their relationship to the QRS.

   • Look before and after the QRS and within the T wave. If you have access to an EKG documenting sinus rhythm, this can be especially helpful in picking out subtle changes.

2. **Find the initiation and termination of the arrhythmia**.

   • Look for a gradual increase or decrease in heart rate and a sudden onset and termination of the arrhythmia.

   • Identify if the rhythm initiates with a premature atrial contraction (PAC) or premature ventricular contraction (PVC).

Adenosine and SVT

A narrow complex rhythm identifies a supraventricular origin that passes through the AV node on its way to the ventricles. Adenosine blocks conduction temporarily in the AV node. Sometimes this will result in termination of the arrhythmia long enough for the sinus node to resume its duty. This is frequently the case in reentrant tachycardias involving the AV node. Less frequently, it can occur in atrial tachycardia. In other cases, adenosine will temporarily block conduction in the AV node, resulting in a brief slowing of the ventricular response. This allows for visualization of underlying atrial activity and can help establish the diagnosis. For example, this can be helpful in distinguishing between a rapid atrial flutter (EKG 9.1) and rapid AV node reentrant tachycardia (EKG 9.2).

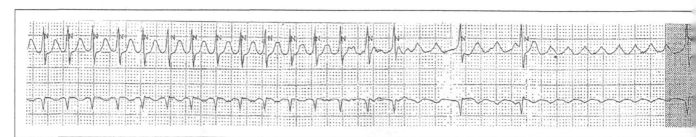

EKG 9.1

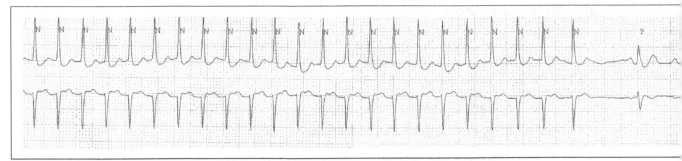

EKG 9.2

Clinical Point: In general, any arrhythmia that terminates with adenosine is likely to be amenable to catheter ablation. Vagal maneuvers are also commonly used in an attempt to slow or break the circuit, as they temporarily slow conduction within the AV node, similar to adenosine. These include bearing down or applying pressure to the carotid artery baroreceptor in the area just below the mandible. This is called carotid sinus massage and is generally avoided in older patients due to the risk of underlying carotid artery disease.

PAROXYSMAL SUPRAVENTRICULAR TACHYCARDIA

SVT can be further classified as **paroxysmal supraventricular tachycardia (PSVT)**. This implies a sudden onset and sudden termination of the arrhythmia. It is generally used in reference to three common types of SVT, all of which present with a regular rhythm. Although this is not all encompassing, the most common types of PSVT encountered in everyday clinical practice are listed below.

• Ectopic atrial tachycardia

• Atrioventricular node reentrant tachycardia (AVNRT)

• Atrioventricular reentrant tachycardia (AVRT)

PSVT can be treated with medications, but radiofrequency ablation is an attractive option given the ability to precisely locate the area of abnormal tissue and the associated high cure rate. Some types of PSVT are more amenable to catheter ablation than others. It is important to be able to recognize these arrhythmias on EKG to provide the best possible patient care.

Ectopic Atrial Tachycardia

Ectopic atrial tachycardia consists of three or more PACs and is defined as sustained if it lasts longer than 30 seconds. In general, ectopic or focal atrial tachycardia occurs via three mechanisms:

- **Enhanced automaticity**, or extreme excitability of the atrial tissue
- **Triggered activity**, such as a catecholamine surge
- **Microreentry**, involving a localized area of excitable tissue that causes multiple premature beats to initiate a tachycardia

Atrial tachycardia involves one focus somewhere in either atrium that overdrive suppresses the sinus node to become the dominant pacemaker (Figure 9.1). At slower rates, a P wave will be evident, but it may have a different morphology than the normal P wave. This depends on the location of the ectopic focus relative to the sinus node. At faster rates, the P wave will be buried in the QRS complex or the T wave, making the definitive diagnosis difficult based on only surface EKG.

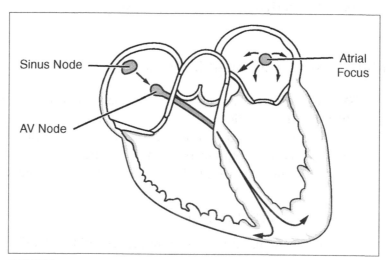

FIGURE 9.1

As the atrial rate increases, the PR interval will gradually prolong, similar to a Wenckebach phenomenon. This occurs because **the faster the AV node is stimulated, the longer its refractory period becomes**. After successive atrial impulses, the P wave becomes buried in the preceding T wave. At faster rates, the P wave may not be identifiable at all. As the atrial rate slows, P waves will become visible again as the PR interval returns to normal prior to termination of the atrial tachycardia (EKG 9.3). This is why it is imperative to examine the initiation and the termination of all SVTs. In this example, an atrial paced beat is seen on termination of the atrial tachycardia before normal sinus rhythm resumes.

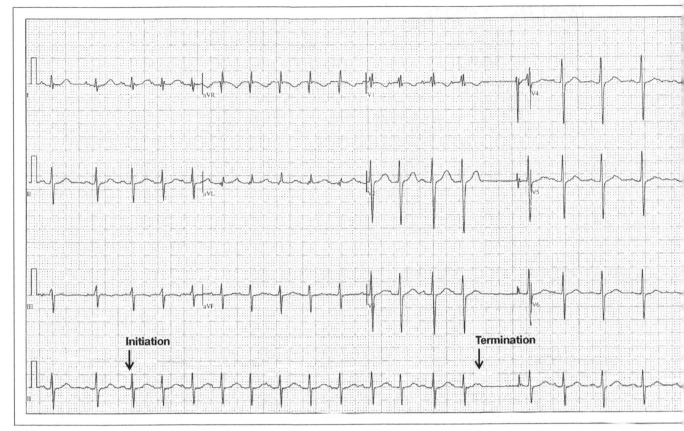

EKG 9.3

Unlike AVNRT and AVRT discussed next, atrial tachycardia is less likely to terminate with adenosine, although it may briefly slow the ventricular response. This is because the AV node does not initiate or sustain the tachycardia as it does in reentrant tachycardias. Atrial tachycardia requires only excitable atrial tissue for its initiation and maintenance.

Atrial tachycardia can occur in both structurally normal and abnormal hearts and is frequently associated with other medical conditions that cause physiologic stress. *Clinical Point*: Common associated conditions include COPD exacerbation, pneumonia, and sepsis. Be careful not to confuse sinus tachycardia with atrial tachycardia. As the term implies, paroxysmal SVT will start suddenly and is often associated with a distinct change in P wave morphology. In sinus tachycardia, the heart rate will gradually increase and the P wave morphology will not change.

REENTRANT TACHYCARDIAS

AVNRT and AVRT are further classified as reentrant tachycardias. By definition, reentrant circuits have two limbs and require three components:

1. Unidirectional block

2. Slow conduction of an impulse

3. Recovery at the block site

These three components will be reviewed in detail for each type of reentrant tachycardia to allow for a full understanding of the mechanism involved in each.

AV Node Reentrant Tachycardia

AVNRT is composed of two types: typical and atypical.

Typical AVNRT

This is the most commonly occurring PSVT. It frequently affects middle-aged patients, although it can occur in any age group. This arrhythmia is the result of a rapidly conducting impulse utilizing two pathways within the AV node.

In typical AVNRT, patients have a dual AV node, consisting of a slow pathway with a fast recovery time and a fast pathway with a slow recovery time. In normal AV nodal function, only the fast pathway is present.

Both of these pathways are able to conduct antegrade from atria to ventricles and retrograde from ventricles to atria. In typical AVNRT, a normal impulse travels down the fast (normal) pathway, which is then slow to recover (repolarize). In the meantime, a PAC arrives early at the fast pathway. It is unable to travel down this pathway because it is still refractory, but it is able to travel down the electrically excitable slow pathway. Once it gets to the end of the slow pathway, the fast pathway is recovered fully and happy to take up the impulse in retrograde fashion. This causes retrograde activation of the atria and sets up a loop tachycardia (Figure 9.2).

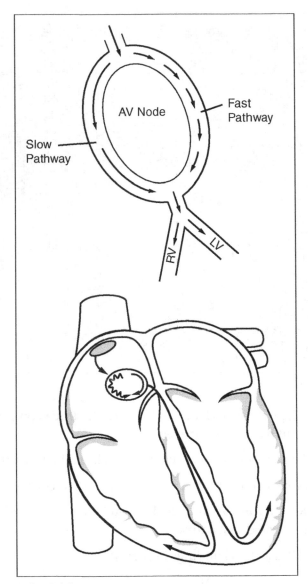

FIGURE 9.2

The ventricles are stimulated antegrade by a PAC via the slow pathway, and the atria are stimulated retrograde by continuation of this impulse via the fast pathway. As a result, electrical activation occurs in the atria and ventricles almost simultaneously, and, therefore, the P waves are buried in the QRS (EKG 9.4). Less commonly, retrograde conduction to the atria is more delayed, and P waves are seen in the terminal portion of the QRS as a pseudo-s wave in II, III, aVF, or a pseudo-r wave in V1, or both.

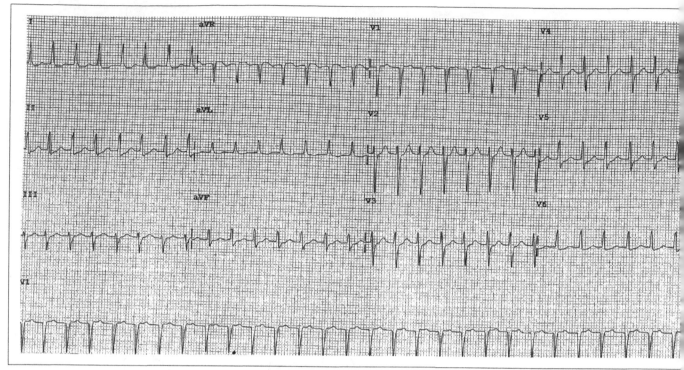

EKG 9.4

Typical AVNRT occurs because the three components necessary for a reentrant circuit have been satisfied:

- *Unidirectional block*: The PAC blocks at the fast pathway.

- *Slow conduction of an impulse*: The PAC is conducted via the slow pathway.

- *Recovery at the block site*: The PAC is conducted retrograde to the atria via the now recovered fast pathway.

Classic EKG findings in typical AVNRT:

- Initiates with PAC

- P wave is buried within the QRS and is usually not visible

- Rarely, the P wave is evident in the terminal portion of the QRS

Clinical Point: When initiation and termination are not available to review, rapid ectopic atrial tachycardia and typical AVNRT can look identical on EKG. In fact, this is a common differential diagnosis, given their electrocardiographic appearance.

Atypical AVNRT

This accounts for only 10% of AVNRT. The electrophysiologic circuits are complex and not as well understood; however, there are two common mechanisms that are generally accepted.

One type of atypical AVNRT involves a reversal of the fast pathway and slow pathway functions. The resultant loop tachycardia is just opposite of that seen in typical AVNRT (Figure 9.2). In these patients, normal conduction travels antegrade to the ventricles via the slow pathway, which conducts slowly and recovers quickly. A PAC arrives early and blocks at the still refractory slow pathway. It races down the fast pathway and is then transmitted retrograde via the quick-to-recover slow pathway. Another type of atypical AVNRT does not utilize a fast pathway but rather involves antegrade conduction via one slow pathway and retrograde conduction via another slow pathway.

Because the atria are stimulated via the slow pathway in both mechanisms, inverted P waves are more likely to be visible on the EKG in the terminal portion of the QRS, because atrial activation will occur slightly later than ventricular activation. On surface EKG, atypical AVNRT can be diagnosed by inverted P waves in the terminal portion of the QRS in leads II, III, and aVF (pseudo-s wave) and V1 (pseudo-r wave) (EKG 9.5).

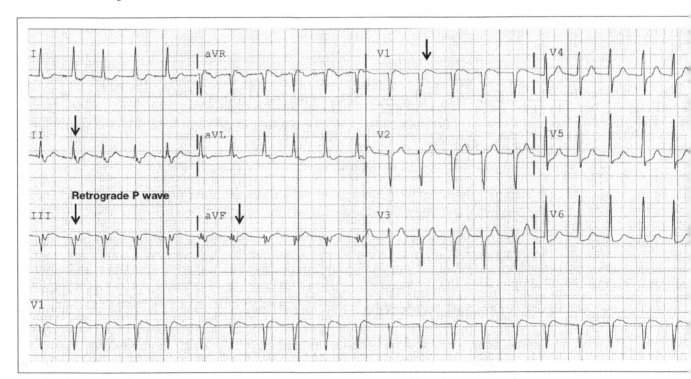

EKG 9.5

The inferior leads reflect activity in the inferior portion of the heart. Recall from Chapter 6 that if electricity is moving away from an area in the heart, it will be reflected by a negative deflection in those particular leads. The often elusive initiation of atypical AVNRT is captured nicely in EKG 9.6. A PAC can be seen buried in a T wave followed by a long PR interval. This depicts the slow conduction of the retrograde impulse to the atria via the slow pathway, setting up the loop tachycardia.

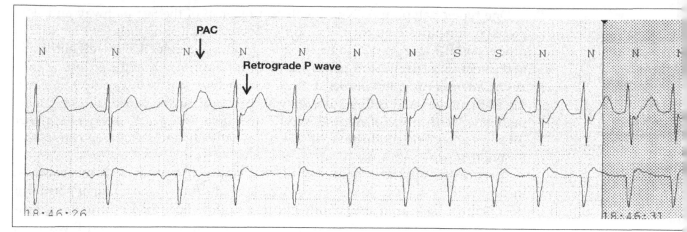

EKG 9.6

Atypical AVNRT occurs because the three components necessary for a reentrant circuit have been satisfied:

- *Unidirectional block*: The PAC blocks at the slow pathway.

- *Slow conduction of an impulse*: The PAC is conducted via the fast pathway (or the second slow pathway if this mechanism is present). The overall conduction is slow because of its initial delay when it is blocked.

- *Recovery at the block site*: The PAC is conducted retrograde to the atria via the slow pathway.

Classic EKG findings in atypical AVNRT:

- Initiates with a PAC. Less commonly a PVC can cause retrograde activation of the atria, initiating the loop tachycardia.

- Retrograde P waves evident in the terminal portion of the QRS in leads II, III, and aVF (pseudo-s waves) and V1 (pseudo-r waves).

Atrioventricular Reentrant Tachycardia

This is also referred to as accessory pathway SVT. AVRT is caused by an area of abnormal conducting tissue outside of the AV node called the bundle of Kent. If this pathway is active and conducts antegrade, a short PR interval (<120 milliseconds or 0.12 seconds) will be visible with a notch in the upstroke of the QRS when the patient is in normal sinus rhythm. This notching in the QRS is called a **delta wave** (EKG 9.7). Electricity spreads from the sinus node down through the bundle of Kent, bypassing the AV node on its way to the ventricles. The combination of a delta wave and a short PR interval is referred to as **pre-excitation** because the ventricles are being stimulated earlier than normal. When pre-excitation is present, the EKG can vary markedly in terms of the delta wave, depending on whether the accessory pathway is lateral, anterior, or posterior. It is usually easiest to see in the precordial leads.

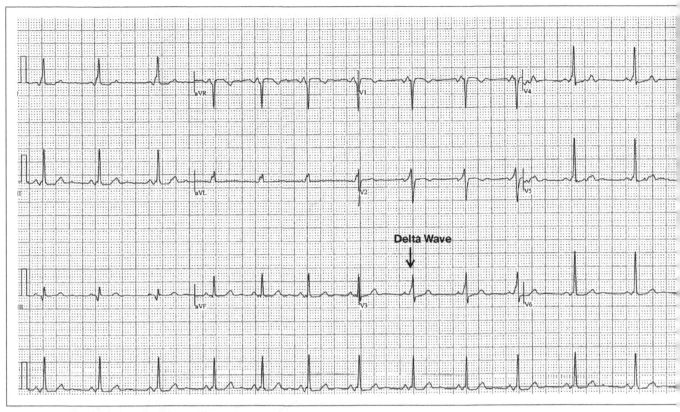

Delta Wave

EKG 9.7

Not all patients will have evidence of this pathway when in normal sinus rhythm. If the patient manifests an SVT but has no evidence of pre-excitation when in sinus rhythm, he or she is said to have a **concealed pathway**. Concealed pathways only conduct retrograde to initiate and maintain the arrhythmia; therefore, no delta wave is present.

When AVRT initiates, it is defined by the direction of electrical conduction over the accessory pathway: **antegrade** (atrium to ventricle) or **retrograde** (from ventricle to atrium). In contrast to AVNRT, there are usually P waves evident, which help aid in the diagnosis. Similar to AVNRT, a premature beat will initiate the arrhythmia.

There are two types of AVRT. The electrical conduction during the tachycardia occurs as follows:

- **Orthodromic AVRT:** Conduction occurs antegrade via the AV node and retrograde via the accessory pathway (Figure 9.3).

- **Antidromic AVRT:** Conduction occurs antegrade via the accessory pathway and retrograde via the AV node (Figure 9.4).

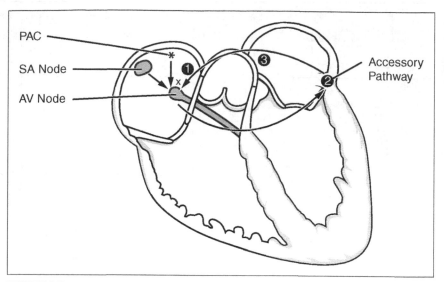

FIGURE 9.3

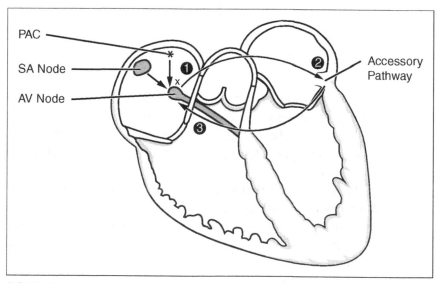

FIGURE 9.4

Orthodromic AVRT

Wolff–Parkinson–White syndrome is a classic example of orthodromic tachy-cardia. In normal sinus rhythm, electrical activity ripples through the atria on its way to the ventricles. The majority of conduction occurs via the accessory

pathway to the ventricles, but just enough electricity is present to slightly depolarize the AV node as well. Antegrade conduction over the accessory pathway
results in a short PR interval and a delta wave. A tachycardia is initiated when a
PAC is unable to conduct via the accessory pathway. The premature beat arrives
while the accessory pathway is still refractory. It is then transmitted via the AV
node in a slower than normal fashion while the AV node continues to repolarize.
By the time this impulse reaches the ventricles, the accessory pathway is fully
recovered and quickly transmits the PAC retrograde to the atria, initiating a loop
tachycardia. On EKG, the delta wave disappears, because the ventricles are now
stimulated via the AV node.

Retrograde P waves are seen in the terminal portion of a narrow QRS in leads
II, III, aVF, and V1, reflective of retrograde atrial activation (EKG 9.8). Recall that a
pathway is said to be concealed if the baseline EKG in normal sinus rhythm does
not exhibit a delta wave. In these patients, the accessory pathway is only able to
conduct retrograde.

Orthodromic tachycardia causes a narrow QRS complex, with a negative P wave
in the terminal portion of the QRS in the inferior leads and lead V1. In orthodromic
tachycardia, the ventricles are still being stimulated via the AV node, so principles
of refractoriness that always apply to the AV node will prevent the ventricular rate
from reaching life-threatening elevations. These patients can be still quite symptomatic from their arrhythmias, and cardiology referral is recommended. As you

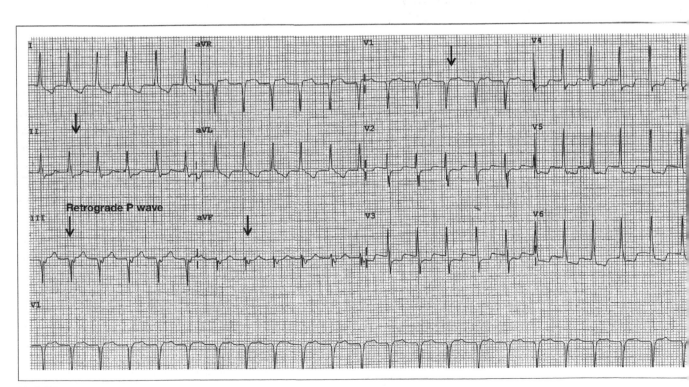

EKG 9.8

might imagine, the EKG of atypical AVNRT and orthodromic AVRT will look almost identical, and electrophysiology studies are often required to make a definitive diagnosis between the two, unless pre-excitation is evident on the EKG when in sinus rhythm.

Orthodromic AVRT occurs because the three components necessary to establish a reentrant circuit have been satisfied:

- *Unidirectional block*: PAC blocks at the accessory pathway.

- *Slow conduction of an impulse*: PAC arrives at the AV node early and is conducted slowly while the AV node repolarizes.

- *Recovery at the block site*: PAC is transmitted retrograde via the accessory pathway to the atria.

    Classic EKG findings in orthodromic AVRT:

- Initiates with a PAC or less commonly a PVC

- Retrograde P waves in the terminal portion of the QRS in the inferior leads (pseudo-s waves) and lead V1 (pseudo-r waves)

- Narrow QRS

- EKG after termination of tachycardia may or may not show pre-excitation. Recall that orthodromic AVRT without evidence of pre-excitation is due to a concealed accessory pathway.

Antidromic AVRT

This form of AVRT is much less common. It is also more dangerous because ventricular stimulation occurs via the unpredictable accessory pathway and not the predictable AV node. In sinus rhythm, normal electrical activation of the ventricles will occur via the AV node or the accessory pathway, depending on which is able to transmit energy faster from the sinus node. If it is transmitted through the accessory pathway, pre-excitation will be evident because the atrial impulse is able to travel faster through the accessory pathway than the AV node on its way to the ventricles.

When tachycardia occurs, it is initiated by a PAC or less commonly by a PVC. Normal electrical activity starts in the sinus node and spreads through the atria to the ventricles. A PAC blocks in the AV node because it is still refractory from the normal beat just prior. It then conducts slowly through the accessory pathway. After it reaches the ventricles, it is transmitted retrograde up the now recovered AV node, initiating the loop tachycardia. It will look distinctly different from orthodromic tachycardia because the ventricles are stimulated outside the AV node, resulting in a wide QRS, which can resemble ventricular tachycardia (EKG 9.9).

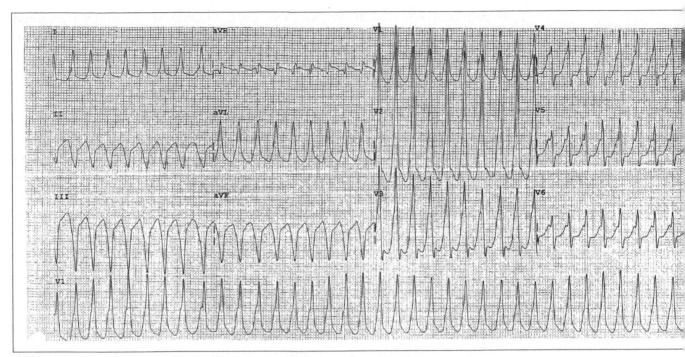

EKG 9.9

Clinical Point: An accessory pathway that can conduct antegrade can be potentially dangerous if a patient develops atrial fibrillation. Unlike the AV node, there are no principles of refractoriness when it comes to the accessory pathway. 1:1 conduction of rapid atrial impulses via the accessory pathway can result in syncope or even death if ventricular fibrillation occurs from such rapid rates.

Antidromic AVRT occurs because the three components necessary to have a reentrant circuit have been satisfied:

- *Unidirectional block*: PAC blocks at the AV node

- *Slow conduction of an impulse*: PAC conducts slowly through the accessory pathway

- *Recovery at the block site*: PAC is transmitted retrograde up the AV node back to the atria

Classic EKG findings in antidromic tachycardia:

- Wide QRS due to ventricular stimulation via the accessory pathway

- Resembles ventricular tachycardia

- EKG after termination will usually have delta waves and evidence of pre-excitation

Clinical Point: If you see a delta wave on an EKG, take a careful history. On the basis of EKG only you cannot determine whether antidromic or orthodromic tachycardia may occur or whether it will ever manifest at all. If the patient has tachypalpitations with near syncope or syncope, a cardiology referral is warranted immediately given the high success rate of radiofrequency ablations and the potential complications of an accessory atrioventricular pathway.

JUNCTIONAL ECTOPIC TACHYCARDIA

Junctional ectopic tachycardia (JET) is not as common as the other types of tachycardias. This is usually the result of overmedication with rate-slowing drugs, or it can occur in the setting of acute inferior wall myocardial infarction. An increased automaticity of the AV node initiates an accelerated junctional rhythm, which resolves once the precipitating event is identified and treated. The EKG will show abnormal appearing or absent P waves with a narrow complex QRS. Frequently, there is evidence of atrioventricular dissociation and inverted P waves. The heart rate is typically 70 to 120 bpm. *Clinical Point*: Digoxin toxicity is a frequent cause of JET.

ATRIAL FIBRILLATION

This is the most common sustained arrhythmia seen worldwide. In atrial fibrillation, there are multiple reentrant circuits present in the atria that propagate impulses in a chaotic fashion. This results in an atrial rate ≥300 bpm due to the extreme excitability of the atrial tissue (Figure 9.5).

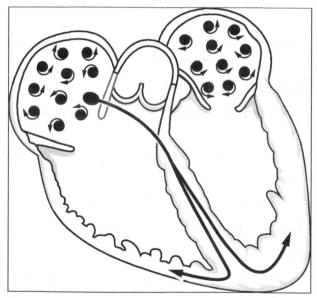

FIGURE 9.5

Atrial activity is seen on an EKG as a wavy, jagged baseline. There are no clear P waves. The conduction slows significantly when these impulses reach the AV node, as it is considerably less excitable than the atrial tissue. As the atrial impulses rapidly penetrate the AV node, it only partially depolarizes. This results in a state of refractoriness that limits the ventricular rate to somewhere usually between 110 and 180 bpm. The rate may be slower in the presence of conduction system disease or medical therapy. It may be faster depending on the overall functionality of the AV node and current physiologic conditions. The resultant QRS complexes are irregular because of the chaotic, disorganized transmission of impulses through the AV node to the ventricles (EKG 9.10).

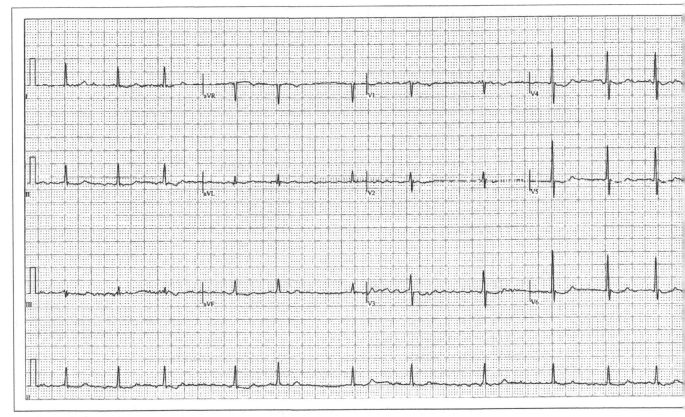

EKG 9.10

The hallmarks of atrial fibrillation are as follows:

- Lack of clear P waves

- Fibrillatory baseline with irregularly irregular QRS complexes

If clinical information is available, atrial fibrillation should be classified based on the length of time the patient has been in the arrhythmia. This involves careful utilization of subjective and objective findings. Paroxysmal atrial fibrillation is defined as periods of sinus rhythm alternating with periods of arrhythmia. Persistent atrial fibrillation has been ongoing without any periods of sinus rhythm for at least 1 week. Patients are said to have entered the chronic phase of atrial fibrillation if maneuvers that maintain sinus rhythm have either failed or been forgone. The term lone atrial fibrillation refers to arrhythmia in the absence of other structural cardiac conditions and hypertension.

Clinical Point: There are four common risk factors that predispose patients to the development of atrial fibrillation:

- Advanced age

- Structural heart disease

- Hypertension

- Obstructive sleep apnea

In general, atrial fibrillation increases the risk of stroke fivefold and, therefore, it is imperative to be able to recognize and diagnose this by EKG. After the diagnosis of atrial fibrillation has been established by EKG, a treatment plan can begin. As part of this, the patient should be assigned a CHADS2 score. This was established using data from the 2001 National Registry of Patients with Atrial Fibrillation.

C: Congestive heart failure: 1 point

H: Hypertension with consistent blood pressure of 140/90 untreated, or treated hypertension: 1 point

A: Age > 75: 1 point

D: Diabetes: 1 point

S2: Stroke or transient ischemic attack: 2 points

This is a general assessment of stroke risk based on the presence of comorbidities, and it will help determine the appropriate level of anticoagulation to initiate (Table 9.1). Each letter stands for a stroke risk factor and, if present, is assigned 1 point. Stroke or transient ischemic attack is assigned 2 points. If the CHADS2 score is ≥2, warfarin or a similar anticoagulant is recommended pending a review of the risk and benefit of anticoagulation. If the CHADS2 score is 0, aspirin is recommended. If the CHADS2 score is 1–2, aspirin or warfarin may be used depending on the overall clinical picture. *Clinical Point*: The risk and benefit of anticoagulation

TABLE 9.1 Stroke Risk with Atrial Fibrillation

CHADS2 Score	Annual CVA Risk (%)	Risk Category	Anticoagulation
≥3	5.3	High	Warfarin or similar anticoagulant
1–2	2.7	Moderate	Aspirin or warfarin
0	0.8	Low	Aspirin

should be always weighed carefully prior to initiation. Take a careful history regarding anemia, history of gastrointestinal or intracranial bleeding, fall risk, and medication noncompliance.

ATRIAL FLUTTER

Atrial flutter is a common arrhythmia that is a form of a macroreentrant atrial circuit. It is more organized than atrial fibrillation and, therefore, has a more regular appearance (EKG 9.11). In atrial flutter, energy is transmitted around a single circuit or several predominant circuits as opposed to numerous circuits as seen in atrial fibrillation (Figure 9.6). Similar to atrial fibrillation, the atrial reentrant circuit rate in atrial flutter is around 300 bpm. Thankfully, the AV node is usually unable to conduct this rapidly in 1:1 fashion. *Clinical Point*: Rapid 1:1 conduction at 300 bpm can be seen in unusual circumstances, such as treatment with a sodium channel blocker.

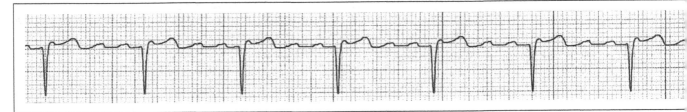

EKG 9.11

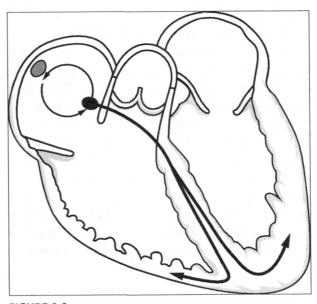

FIGURE 9.6

Most commonly the AV node will conduct every two or three impulses from the atrial flutter circuit, resulting in a ventricular rate that is a function of 300 bpm. If there is 2:1 flutter, the ventricular rate will be 150 bpm. In other words, for every two atrial impulses, there is one ventricular impulse. If there is 3:1 flutter, the ventricular rate will be 100 bpm. 4:1 flutter results in a ventricular rate of 75 bpm. Flutter rates can be even slower in the presence of conduction disease or rate-slowing medications that would further delay conduction through the AV node. Flutter rates may also be described as variable, which results from less predictability in the conduction through the AV node. For instance, the flutter circuit may vary from 3:1 to 4:1 at times, resulting in a rhythm that may be slightly irregular even though there is a sawtooth P wave pattern seen.

Atrial flutter can be difficult to distinguish from other atrial arrhythmias when it occurs at faster rates, such as greater than 150 bpm. It is important to look for subtle nuances on the EKG that can aid in the diagnosis. Initiation, termination, and breaks or pauses in the rhythm are extremely helpful. Vagal maneuvers or adenosine can be attempted as well. These are unlikely to terminate atrial flutter but may slow conduction through the AV node just long enough so that you can identify flutter waves in between QRS complexes.

There are two types of atrial flutter. It is imperative to make the distinction between the two as the treatment can vary greatly:

- Typical atrial flutter

- Atypical atrial flutter

Typical Atrial Flutter

Typical or counterclockwise atrial flutter originates from a single circuit localized in the right atrium around the tricuspid valve. It is easy to spot because it has a "typical," reproducible pattern on 12-lead EKG.

The electrical circuit transmits energy in a counterclockwise fashion around the tricuspid valve. Picture a clock face around the tricuspid annulus (Figure 9.7). Now superimpose a 12-lead EKG over it. Typical atrial flutter can be diagnosed on EKG by negative P waves in the inferior leads II, III, and aVF and positive P waves in V1 (EKG 9.12). Less commonly clockwise typical flutter may be present. This utilizes the same circuit, but it transmits energy the opposite way, resulting in positive P waves in leads II, III, and aVF and negative P waves in V1 (EKG 9.13). *Clinical Point*: It is important to be able to recognize typical flutter, as it carries a high cure rate by radiofrequency ablation.

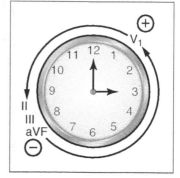

FIGURE 9.7

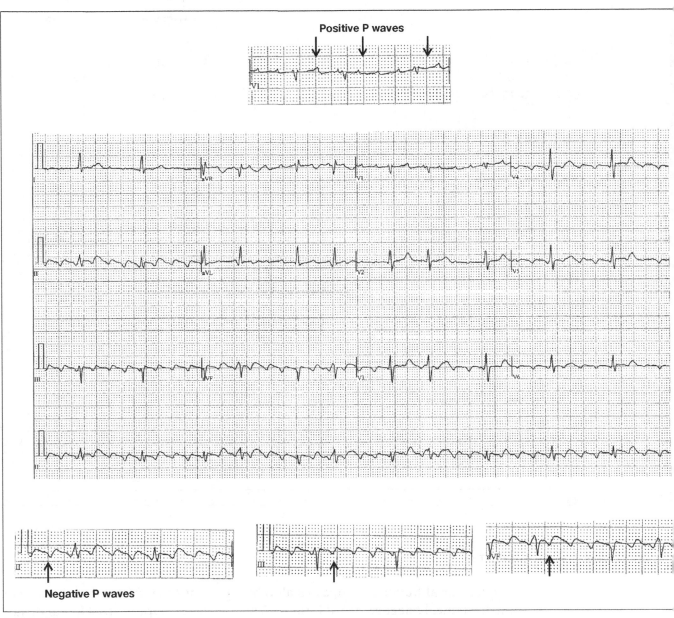

Positive P waves

Negative P waves

EKG 9.12

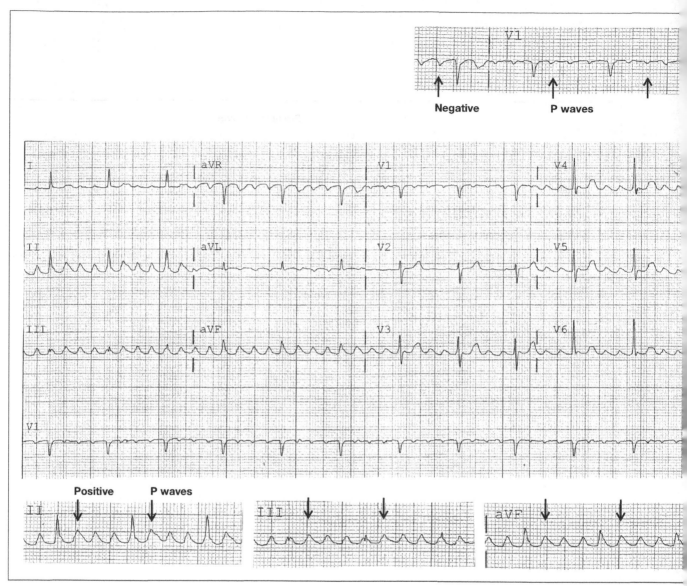

EKG 9.13

Atypical Atrial Flutter

Atypical atrial flutter encompasses all other types of atrial flutter that do not fall into the typical category by EKG criteria. The P waves in atypical atrial flutter do not follow a particular pattern because there is usually more than one macroreentrant circuit present (EKG 9.14). Because of this, atypical atrial flutter tends to be more difficult to treat by radiofrequency ablation and sometimes antiarrhythmic or rate control medications will be attempted first. The same sawtooth pattern is present reflecting rapid atrial conduction representative of the dominant flutter circuit.

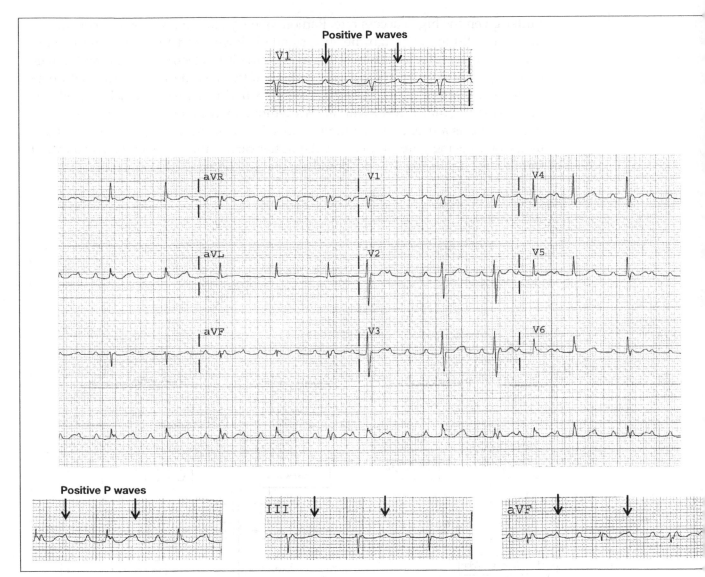

EKG 9.14

Clinical Point: Atrial flutter does not usually occur in otherwise structurally normal hearts. It is a common complication of valvular heart disease, myocardial infarction, uncontrolled hypertension, pulmonary disease, and obstructive sleep apnea. It can also occur following open heart surgery.

Treatment of Atrial Flutter

There are many treatment options for both typical and atypical flutter. Electrophysiology study and radiofrequency ablation are attractive treatment options for typical flutter given the high success rate. Radiofrequency ablation can also be considered in atypical flutter, although the success rate is lower, and the procedure is more involved as there is usually more than one circuit to electrically map and ablate. Other options for both typical and atypical flutter include rate control with beta blockers, calcium channel blockers, and digoxin; direct current synchronized cardioversion; rhythm control with antiarrhythmic medications; or even rapid atrial pacing. This is a useful option in post–open heart surgical patients who still have temporary pacing wires in place. Atrial flutter carries the same stroke risk as atrial fibrillation, and these patients should also be assigned a CHADS2 score.

REVIEW OF SVT

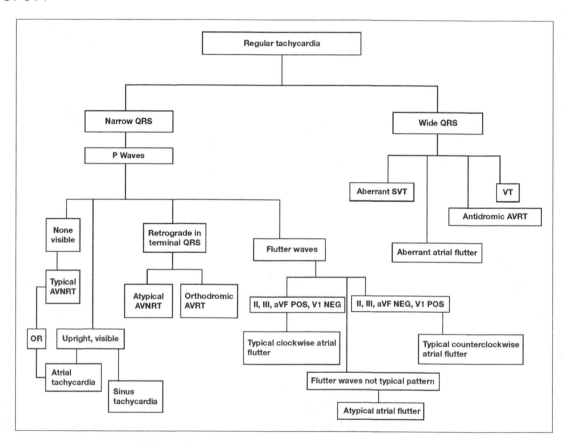

Similar Appearing PSVT on EKG

1. Rapid atrial tachycardia and typical AVNRT: P wave buried in preceding T wave

2. Orthodromic AVRT and atypical AVNRT: Inverted P wave in inferior leads and lead V1

CHAPTER 9 REVIEW QUESTIONS

1. Typical AVNRT is composed of a _____ and a _____ pathway.

2. Atrial fibrillation is defined by a lack of _____ waves and QRS complexes that are _____.

3. P waves in typical counterclockwise atrial flutter are _____ in leads II, III, aVF, and _____ in V1.

4. The presence of a delta wave and a short PR interval is termed _____.

5. In orthodromic tachycardia, the ventricles are stimulated via the _____.

6. In antidromic tachycardia, the ventricles are stimulated via the _____.

7. A CHADS2 score should be assigned to patients with atrial fibrillation and atrial flutter to help assess their risk of _____.

Ventricular Arrhythmias

INTRODUCTION

There are three main arrhythmias that can arise from the ventricles, ranging from benign to life threatening. These include the following:

- Premature ventricular contractions (PVCs)
- Ventricular tachycardia (VT)
- Ventricular fibrillation (VF)

It is up to the clinician to be able to recognize clues available on a 12-lead EKG in addition to other clinical factors to establish a diagnosis and guide the treatment plan.

PREMATURE VENTRICULAR CONTRACTIONS

PVCs are easily recognized because they originate in the ventricles rather than the atria and therefore do not follow the normal conduction pathway. Because of this, they have a completely different appearance from normal beats and PACs. When a focus becomes irritable and initiates an impulse, the stimulus starts somewhere in the ventricles and spreads through the surrounding myocardium aberrantly (Figure 10.1). This results in a wide-appearing QRS complex (EKG 10.1). The T wave of each PVC will sometimes point in the opposite direction from the QRS, and PVCs are often accompanied by a compensatory pause. Although PVCs are commonly a benign finding, they generally warrant further investigation. They can be a clue that there is irritability of the ventricular myocardium, possibly secondary to underlying ischemia.

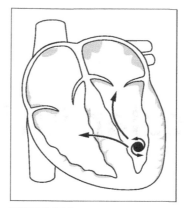

FIGURE 10.1

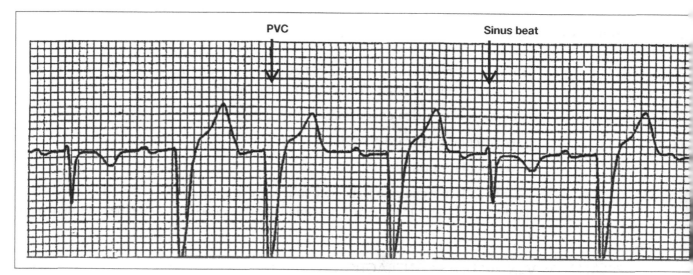

EKG 10.1

There are two reasons to treat PVCs: (1) they are potentially life threatening and (2) they cause lifestyle-limiting symptoms. The following are factors that should always be noted with regard to PVCs:

• Unifocal versus multifocal appearance

• Symptomatic or asymptomatic nature

• Frequency of PVCs

• Presence or absence of structural cardiac abnormalities

PVCs can be isolated or occur in pairs, called ventricular couplets. If every other beat is premature, this is referred to as ventricular bigeminy (EKG 10.2). If every third beat is premature, this is referred to as ventricular trigeminy (EKG 10.3).

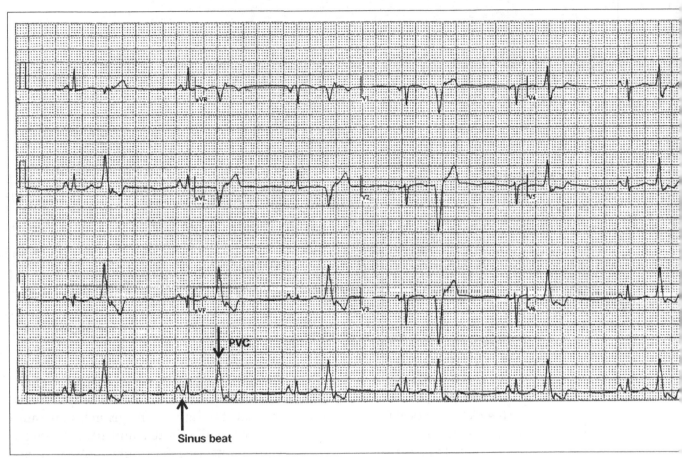

EKG 10.2

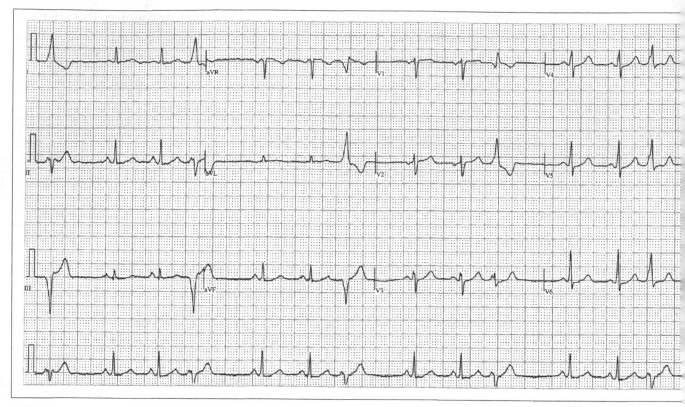

EKG 10.3

PVCs should be described as unifocal or multifocal, which refers to the appearance of the PVC. Unifocal PVCs will appear the same throughout any given lead because they arise from the same site within the ventricle (EKGs 10.2 and 10.3). These are more likely to be benign and commonly arise from the left or right ventricular out-flow tract. *Clinical Point*: Multifocal PVCs will have a different appearance from each other in the same lead and in general carry a worse prognosis (EKG 10.4). They are more likely to be associated with structural heart disease.

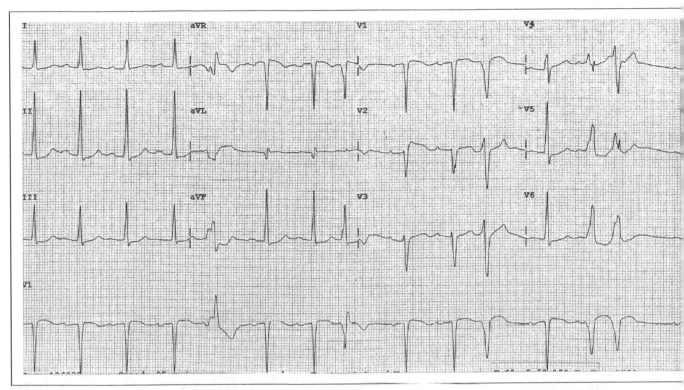

EKG 10.4

VENTRICULAR TACHYCARDIA

A run of three or more consecutive PVCs is termed VT. VT involves a macroreentrant circuit around abnormal tissue in the ventricle, such as scar tissue from a previous myocardial infarction or weakened tissue in the setting of a nonischemic cardiomyopathy (Figure 10.2). VT should be classified as sustained or nonsustained. Sustained VT lasts for greater than 30 seconds. VT is defined by atrioventricular dissociation. The atrial and ventricular impulses occur independently of one another, and there is no identifiable relationship between P waves and QRS complexes. The ventricular rate is almost always faster than the atrial rate, usually between 120 and 200 bpm. If the ventricular rate is very rapid, P waves can be difficult to see (EKG 10.5). Carefully examine each lead. If atrioventricular dissociation can be identified, this is diagnostic of VT. In EKG 10.6, P waves can be easily seen that are dissociated from the QRS complex. AV dissociation can also be noted in EKGs 10.7 and 10.13.

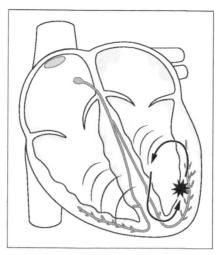

FIGURE 10.2

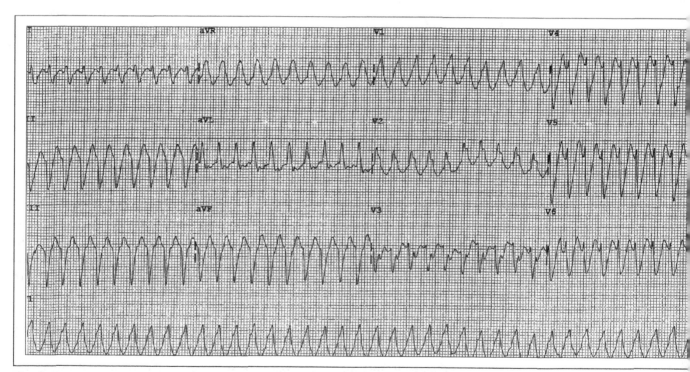

EKG 10.5

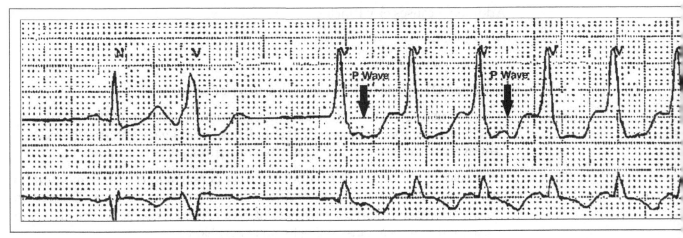

EKG 10.6

Accelerated Idioventricular Rhythm

An accelerated idioventricular rhythm involves a ventricular focus that is faster than a typical junctional rhythm but slower than what is classified as VT, usually falling between 70 and 100 bpm (EKG 10.7). Because of its slower rate, it will compete with the normal sinus mechanism, which will eventually overdrive suppress and terminate it. *Clinical Point*: An accelerated idioventricular rhythm is most commonly seen during acute myocardial infarction or after reperfusion therapy.

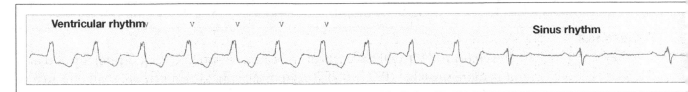

EKG 10.7

Causes of Ventricular Tachycardia

VT most commonly occurs as a complication of ischemic heart disease or left ventricular dysfunction from nonischemic causes, and is frequently seen in the setting of acute myocardial infarction. The arrhythmia may resolve once the initial insult improves, such as after revascularization. If infarction is present, areas of scar in the ventricle can serve as a substrate for VT that occurs as a result of electrical reentry around weakened tissue.

Whether due to nonischemic or ischemic causes, a left ventricular ejection fraction ≤35% places a patient at significantly increased risk for life-threatening ventricular arrhythmias. *Clinical Point*: In the setting of decompensated heart failure, the risk of arrhythmogenic death is even higher.

Additional causes of VT include

- Increased automaticity

- Electrolyte abnormalities

- Prolonged QT interval, which can be primary or acquired

  - Primary long QT syndrome is genetic, whereas acquired long QT syndrome is due to medications such as certain antibiotics, antifungals, antiarrhythmics, or antipsychotic medications. This will be further reviewed in Chapter 12.

VT should always be classified as monomorphic or polymorphic. **Monomorphic VT** will have a repetitive similar appearance with all beats looking the same. This reflects electrical macroreentry around one area of weakened myocardium. In EKG 10.8, a normal rhythm is seen transitioning to monomorphic VT.

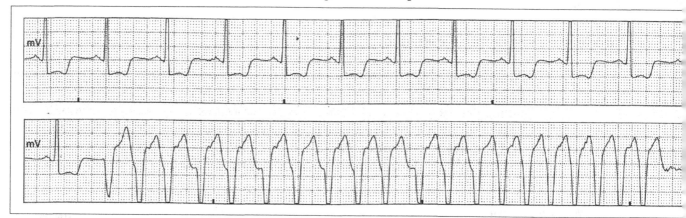

EKG 10.8

Polymorphic VT will have a beat-to-beat variation in QRS morphology and axis and is more unstable (EKG 10.9). This indicates that there is more than one area of irritability within the myocardium.

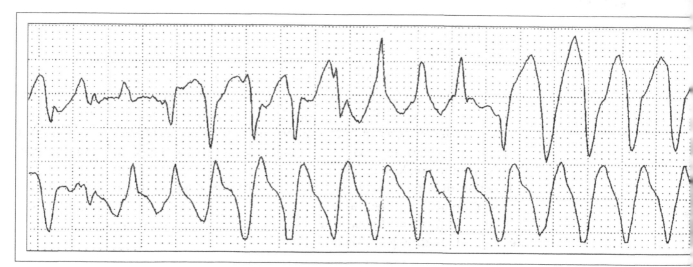

EKG 10.9

Torsades de pointes, or twisting of the points, is a form of polymorphic VT that is particularly unstable. If this type of VT is not terminated, it can quickly degenerate into VF. Torsades is defined by a cyclic rotating of the QRS complexes around the electrical baseline, pointing up or down for a few beats and then twisting in the opposite direction (EKG 10.10). Torsades is most commonly seen in the setting of a prolonged QT interval. Frequent causes include genetic variations; medications; and electrolyte abnormalities such as hypokalemia.

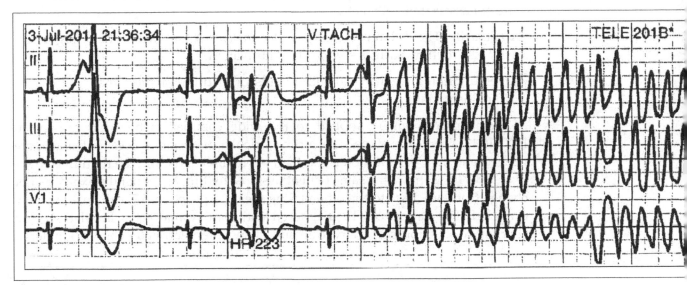

EKG 10.10

VT is life threatening if it is sustained, as patients are not able to maintain an adequate blood pressure due to rapid inefficient ventricular contraction. If VT is not self-terminating, it accelerates and progresses to VF with subsequent sudden cardiac death.

VENTRICULAR TACHYCARDIA VERSUS ABERRANT SVT

VT can be difficult to distinguish from aberrantly conducted supraventricular arrhythmias. When tachycardia occurs in the setting of underlying conduction disease, the QRS duration is wide, causing an unstable appearance. Patients may sometimes develop a rate-related bundle branch block, which causes a wide-appearing QRS during a regular tachycardia.

If a patient has known structural heart disease, especially with left ventricular dysfunction, a wide complex tachycardia should be treated as VT until proven otherwise. VT is much more common than SVT with aberrancy. Many years ago, criteria were established by Wellens, Bar, and Lie (1978) to help distinguish between ventricular arrhythmias and SVT with aberrancy on EKG. When present, these findings are suggestive of VT; however, their absence does not rule out VT.

- **Positive/negative concordance** in all precordial leads: The general QRS direction should be the same in all precordial leads, either negative or positive. A negative concordance is more strongly associated with VT.

- **Indeterminate axis**: The axis is calculated between −90 and +180 degrees.

- The VT axis should be distinctly different than the axis when in normal sinus rhythm. If possible, obtain a previous EKG.

- **A-V dissociation**: Carefully examine each lead and try to identify P waves that are not associated with a QRS.

- **Regularity**: The R-R interval during VT is fairly constant, without an irregularly irregular rhythm, such as seen in atrial fibrillation.

- **QRS duration** more than 140 milliseconds, or RS duration more than 120 milliseconds.

These criteria can be applied to the wide complex tachycardia present in EKG 10.11. There is no evidence of atrioventricular dissociation because P waves are not evident, the QRS duration is less than 140 milliseconds, and the rhythm is irregular. EKG 10.12 shows the same patient in sinus rhythm. Note that the axis does not change from one EKG to the other. Using the criteria above, VT can be effectively excluded. The patient can be diagnosed with paroxysmal atrial fibrillation with aberrant conduction, secondary to an underlying interventricular conduction delay.

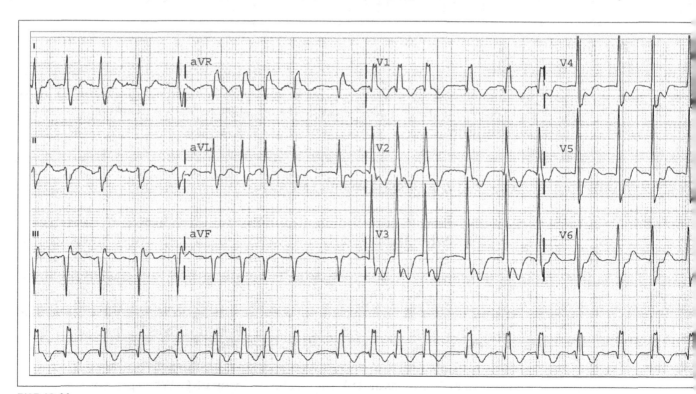

EKG 10.11

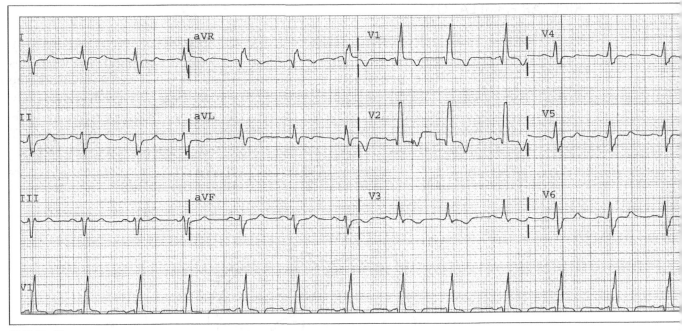

EKG 10.12

Fusion beats are strongly suggestive of VT. A fusion beat occurs when an atrial impulse is transmitted through the atrioventricular node to activate the ventricles at the same time as ventricular depolarization occurs via the ectopic focus generating VT. The two beats converge, causing a more narrow QRS complex than the other surrounding beats (EKG 10.13). Fusion beats are more commonly seen in slower VT as opposed to rapid VT.

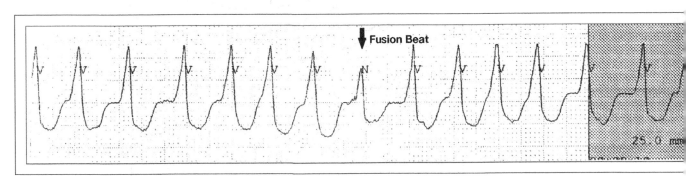

EKG 10.13

VENTRICULAR FIBRILLATION

In contrast to VT, in VF, there is no organized activity in the ventricles (Figure 10.3). The EKG pattern has no identifiable P, QRS, or T wave (EKG 10.14). The ventricles fibrillate inefficiently without meaningful cardiac output. Patients will become unconscious, and unsynchronized direct current shock is indicated immediately on recognition of VF. VF frequently occurs in the setting of cardiac arrest, and it is unlikely to occur in the absence of known structural heart disease or prolonged QT interval. *Clinical Point*: Intravenous amiodarone and/or lidocaine is usually administered to reduce ventricular irritability, as recurrence of VF is common during the same presentation. In patients with sudden cardiac death, VF is the common cause.

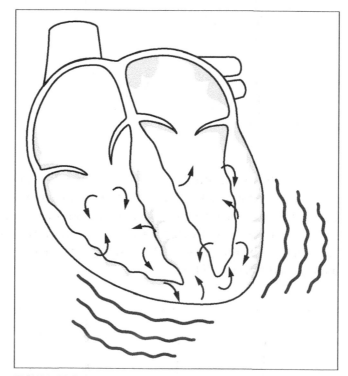

FIGURE 10.3

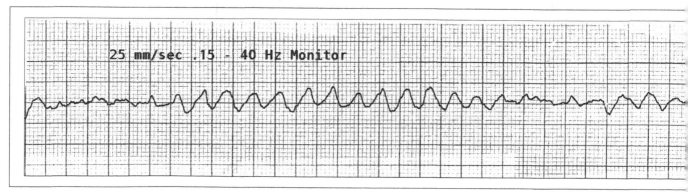

25 mm/sec .15 - 40 Hz Monitor

EKG 10.14

ASYSTOLE

Asystole, or cardiac standstill, is a complete cessation of electrical activity within the heart (EKG 10.15). It is the result of severe tissue hypoxemia and ultimately leads to patient death. Untreated VF will lead to asystole.

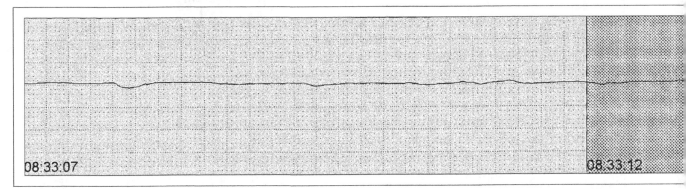

08:33:07   08:33:12

EKG 10.15

BRUGADA PATTERN

A Brugada pattern is a rare but important pattern to look for on EKG. Carefully examine leads V1 to V3. If a Brugada pattern is present, there is an RSR' pattern mimicking an incomplete right bundle branch block with concomitant ST segment elevation (EKG 10.16). The clinical manifestation of this is sudden cardiac death from VF in patients with structurally normal hearts. According to Braunwald (2001), this is thought to be due to a mutation in a cardiac sodium channel and is a genetic defect similar to that which causes long QT syndrome. *Clinical Point*: If a patient has a family history of sudden cardiac death or if they complain of syncope or near syncope, carefully examine leads V1 to V3 for a Brugada pattern.

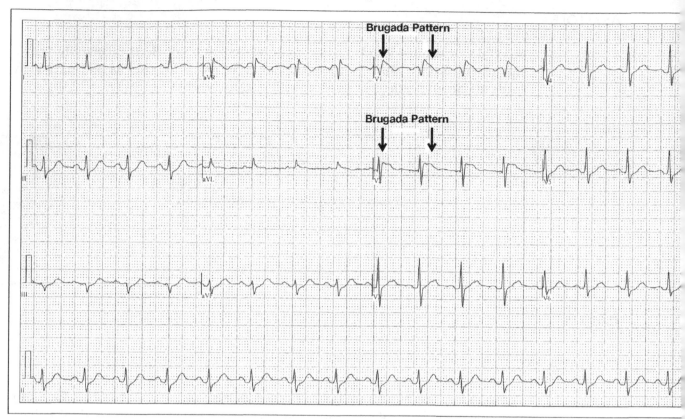

EKG 10.16

CHAPTER 10 REVIEW QUESTIONS

1. In a wide complex tachycardia, _____ is diagnostic of VT.

2. VT that has a repetitive, similar appearance from beat to beat is classified as _____.

3. Polymorphic VT in the setting of a prolonged QT interval is referred to as _____.

4. A complete lack of organized activity in the ventricles is the definition of _____.

5. VF should be treated immediately with _____.

6. _____ PVCs are more likely to be associated with structural heart disease.

7. A wide complex tachycardia in a patient with structural heart disease should be treated as _____ until proven otherwise.

11

Paced EKGs

INTRODUCTION

Paced EKGs are often a confusing topic. The ability of the clinician to interpret a paced EKG is vital, as it is the best tool available in everyday practice to observe for proper function of the pacemaker or implantable cardioverter defibrillator (ICD). It is invaluable in correlating clinical findings to normal or abnormally functioning devices.

Pacemakers are implanted to improve morbidity that is associated with abnormally slow heart rates that cause a decrease in cardiac output and put a patient at risk for bodily injury or death. They also allow for appropriate medical treatment of tachyarrhythmias or ischemic heart disease if there are periods of bradycardia that may limit optimal medical therapy. In general, pacemakers are indicated to treat:

- Bradyarrhythmias

- Syncope and near syncope

- Lifestyle limiting impairment in sinus node response to activity, or, chronotropic incompetence

Pacemakers will not prevent ventricular arrhythmias, whereas ICDs will perform functions to prevent sudden cardiac death from ventricular arrhythmias. Pacemakers are generally indicated to improve morbidity, whereas ICDs improve mortality. All ICDs are also pacemakers and, therefore, all of the information regarding paced rhythms in this chapter will apply to both pacemakers and ICDs. Specific EKG findings regarding ICDs will be reviewed separately. Indications for ICDs are beyond the scope of this book.

INDICATIONS FOR PACEMAKERS

The specific indications for permanent pacemakers are presented in a joint publication by the American College of Cardiology, American Heart Association, and North American Society of Pacing and Electrophysiology. These indications are further classified based on the severity of the conduction disease and presence or absence of symptoms.

Class I indication: Conditions for which there is evidence and/or general agreement that a given procedure or treatment is beneficial.

- Sinus node dysfunction with documented symptomatic bradycardia or chronotropic incompetence

- Symptomatic bradycardia with complete heart block or advanced second-degree atrioventricular (AV) block

- Asymptomatic complete heart block with heart rate less than 40 bpm or periods of asystole lasting greater than 3 seconds

- Fascicular block with intermittent complete heart block or second-degree type II AV block

- Alternating left bundle branch block and right bundle branch block

- Recurrent syncope caused by carotid sinus stimulation

- Pauses greater than 3 seconds induced by minimal carotid sinus pressure

Class II indication: Conditions for which there is conflicting evidence and/or a divergence of opinion about the usefulness of a procedure or treatment.

Class IIa indication: Weight of evidence or opinion is in favor of usefulness.

- Sinus node dysfunction with heart rate less than 40 bpm but no clear association between symptoms and bradycardia

- Syncope and sinus node dysfunction diagnosed by electrophysiology study

- Asymptomatic second-degree type II AV block with narrow QRS or complete heart block with heart rate greater than 40 bpm

- Asymptomatic infranodal block on electrophysiology study

- First- or second-degree AV block with symptoms attributable to AV dyssynchrony

- Syncope not proven to be due to AV block when other likely causes have been excluded

- Incidental finding at electrophysiology study of His-to-ventricle (HV) interval greater than 100 ms

- Recurrent syncope of unclear origin associated with a hypersensitive carotid response

Class IIb indication: Usefulness is less established by evidence or opinion.

- Markedly prolonged PR interval with left ventricular dysfunction and congestive heart failure

- Neuromuscular disease with any degree of AV block or fascicular block with or without symptoms

Class III indication: Conditions for which there is evidence and/or a general agreement that a procedure is not useful or effective and in some cases may be harmful.

- Sinus bradycardia with symptoms due to nonessential drug therapy

- First-degree AV block, asymptomatic second-degree type I AV block, or AV block expected to resolve

- Asymptomatic fascicular block

- Fascicular block with prolonged PR interval without symptoms

- Syncope in the absence of a cardioinhibitory response

- Hyperactive cardioinhibitory response to carotid sinus stimulation when no symptoms or vague symptoms are present

- Situational vasovagal syncope in which avoidance behavior is effective

ANATOMY OF THE PACEMAKER SYSTEM

Pacemaker wires are implanted via the subclavian vein and reside in the right atrium and right ventricle. Pacemakers can be single chamber and pace and sense in the right atrium or right ventricle; dual chamber and pace and sense in the right atrium and right ventricle; or biventricular and pace and sense in the right atrium, right and left ventricle (Figures 11.1–11.3). The indications for each are beyond the scope of this book.

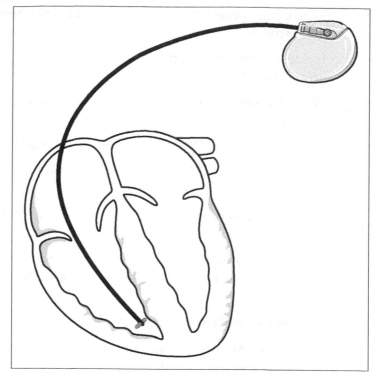

FIGURE 11.1

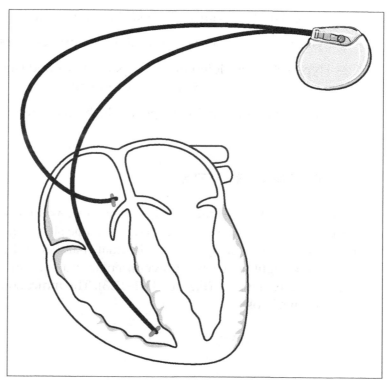

FIGURE 11.2

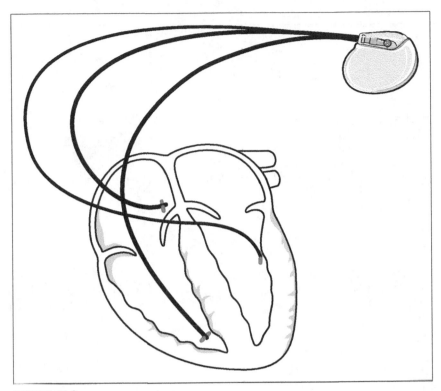

FIGURE 11.3

Pacemaker Leads

There are two types of pacing leads: **unipolar** and **bipolar**. Unipolar leads transmit energy through a larger circuit from the tip of the lead back to the pacemaker generator. Because the electricity covers a larger surface area, it causes a larger pacemaker spike on the surface EKG (EKG 11.1). There is also a greater chance of pectoral muscle stimulation with this configuration. Bipolar leads transmit energy through a smaller circuit, as both poles are located at the tip of the lead. This configuration produces a smaller pacemaker spike on surface EKG (EKG 11.2). In fact, it is not uncommon for bipolar leads to not cause a visible pacing spike at all. Most modern pacemakers are programmed to the bipolar setting, unless improved function is noted in the unipolar setting.

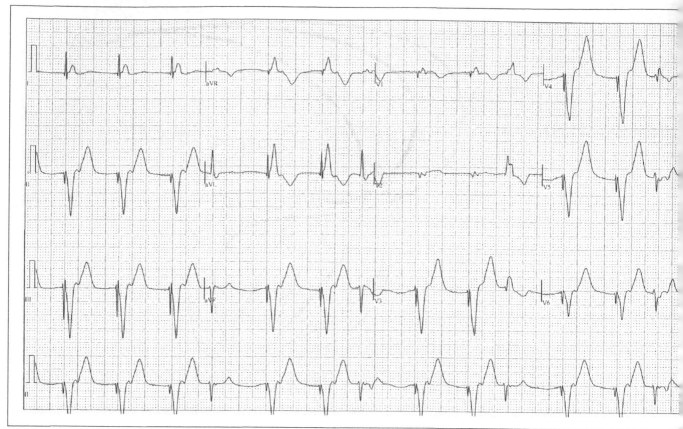

EKG 11.1

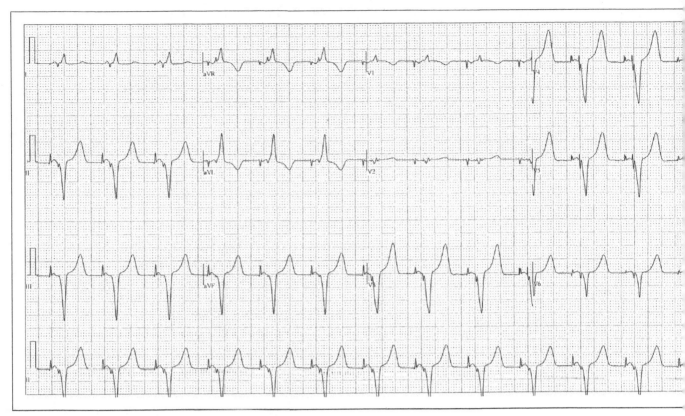

EKG 11.2

ATRIAL PACING

Atrial pacing results in a pacing spike just before a P wave with a slightly different P wave morphology than that seen when intrinsic sinus node activity is present (EKG 11.3). The closer the atrial pacing wire is to the sinus node, the more similar the P waves will be. Atrial pacing will occur if the sinus node fails to pace at the lower rate setting, usually 60 bpm in a pacemaker. *Clinical Point*: Always check the lower pacing rate of the device before assuming there is failure to pace.

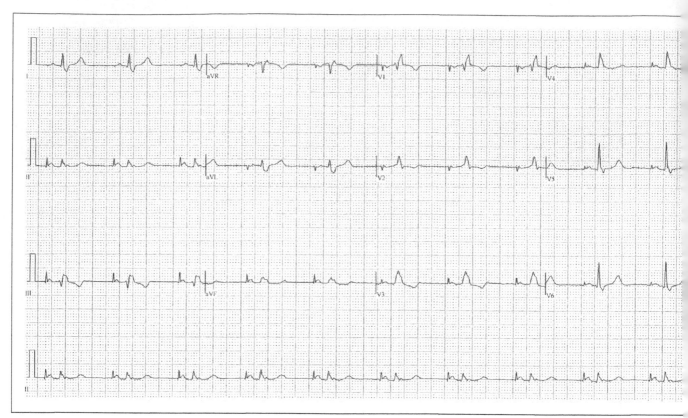

EKG 11.3

VENTRICULAR PACING

Ventricular pacing results in a pacing spike followed by a wide QRS with a left bundle branch block type pattern (EKG 11.4). Ventricular paced beats will have a distinctly different appearance from intrinsic ventricular beats. The right ventricular pacing wire stimulates the right bundle branch first, and the left bundle branch is activated later. This results in a left bundle branch block pattern. As reviewed in Chapter 7, a left bundle branch block pattern creates difficulty in interpreting the EKG for ischemia, whether there is an intrinsic left bundle branch block or whether it is due to right ventricular pacing. If ischemia or infarction is suspected and the patient is not pacemaker dependent, it may be useful to temporarily inhibit ventricular pacing to obtain a 12-lead EKG. In patients with ICDs, the lower pacing rate is often set slower than in pacemaker patients to minimize frequent right ventricular pacing, which may worsen underlying congestive heart failure and cardiomyopathy in these patients.

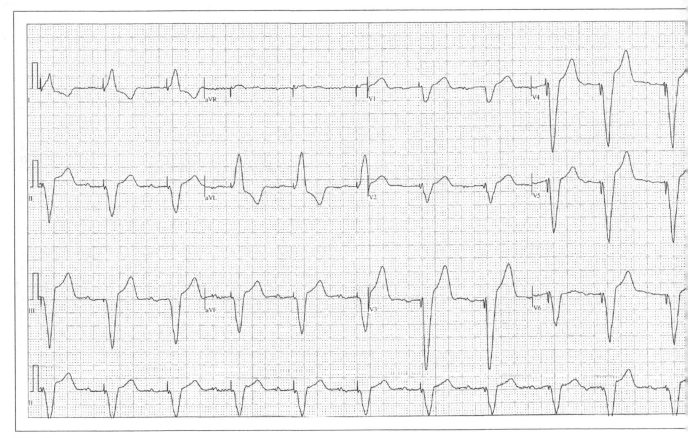

EKG 11.4

DUAL-CHAMBER PACING

Dual-chamber pacing requires a right atrial and a right ventricular lead. Dual-chamber systems are common, as they allow for AV synchrony and thus provide the most physiologic response to normal activities. In EKG 11.5, atrial and ventricular pacing spikes are seen before each P wave and QRS complex. Carefully examine each lead, as pacing spikes will be easier to see in some leads than others.

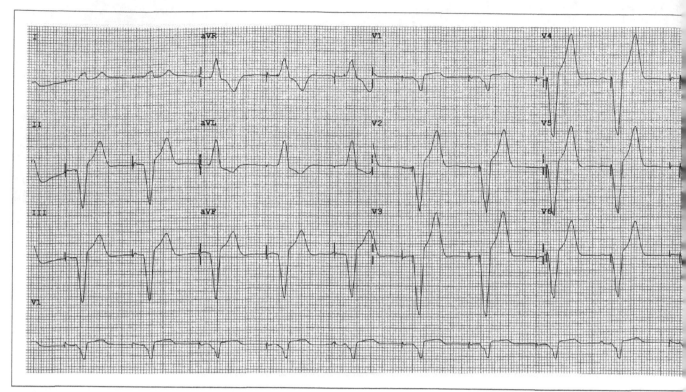

EKG 11.5

BIVENTRICULAR PACING

Biventricular pacing can improve both subjective and objective findings in patients who meet several criteria:

- Advanced heart failure symptoms

- Left bundle branch block on baseline EKG

- Significant left ventricular dysfunction

Patients who meet these criteria often do not do well long term due to an impairment in left ventricular function and dyssynchrony of the ventricles due to a left bundle branch block. By placing a wire in the left ventricle in addition to the right ventricle, both ventricles can be stimulated to beat together. This resynchronization can result in an improvement in left ventricular function and in symptoms of congestive heart failure.

With biventricular pacing, the goal is to achieve pacing as close to 100% of the time as possible. These patients should be followed up closely after implantation.

EKGs and symptoms should be monitored frequently. If there is appropriate pacing in both ventricles, the QRS duration in the postoperative EKG should be more narrow than on the preoperative EKG. Compare the preoperative QRS duration in EKG 11.6 with that of the postoperative EKG 11.7.

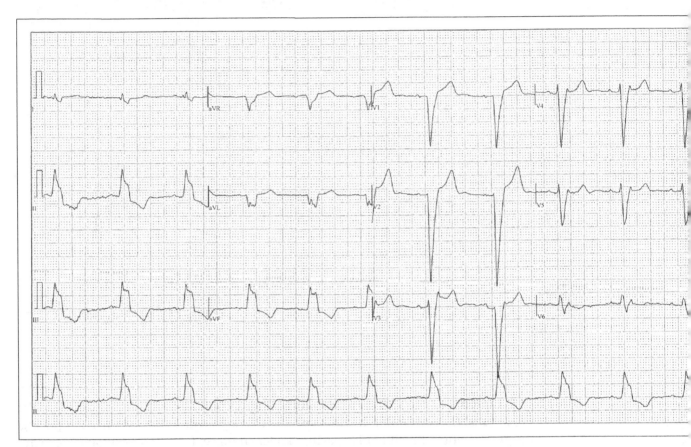

EKG 11.6

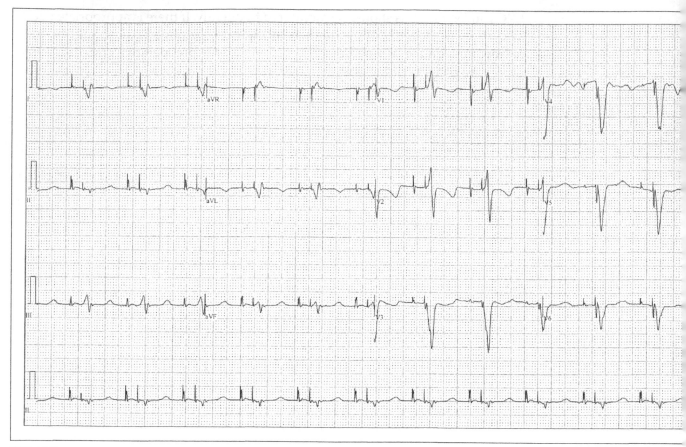

EKG 11.7

Symptoms of congestive heart failure should gradually improve in the majority of patients. *Clinical Point*: If it is suspected that a patient is not biventricular pacing despite having a biventricular pacing device in place, further investigation is warranted. This could be due to lead malfunction, lack of optimal AV synchrony, or inadequate rate control that exceeds the ability of the device to appropriately pace. Less commonly, patients are simply nonresponders to resynchronization therapy.

PACEMAKER MODES

Pacemakers are programmed to sense intrinsic activity and either deliver a pace or inhibit pacing. Pacemaker modes consist of a three- to four-letter description that summarizes the pacing, sensing, and rate responsiveness of the device. The mode is programmed based on the patient's indication for pacing and his or her specific type of pacemaker. These modes are different for single- and dual-chamber pacemakers (Table 11.1).

- *Position 1*: Chamber being paced.
  V = ventricle, A = atrium, D = dual, O = neither

- *Position 2*: Chamber being sensed.
  V = ventricle, A = atrium, D = dual, O = neither

- *Position 3*: Pacing response to a sensed beat.
  I = inhibited, T = triggered, D = dual (inhibited or triggered pace), O = neither

- *Position 4*: Rate response.
  R = rate responsive, O = no rate response

TABLE 11.1 Pacemaker Modes

Position 1	Position 2	Position 3	Position 4
Chamber being paced	Chamber being sensed	Pacing response to a sensed beat	Rate response or lack thereof
V: Ventricle	V: Ventricle	I: Inhibited	R: Rate responsive
A: Atrium	A: Atrium	T: Triggered	O: None (usually blank)
D: Dual (both)	D: Dual (both)	D: Dual—Inhibited or triggered, depending on the chamber	
O: No pacing	O: No sensing	O: Neither	

For example, **DDDR** is a common pacing mode. Based on Table 11.1, this mode indicates that the pacemaker has the ability to pace and sense in the atrium and ventricle. It will respond to a sensed beat in either chamber with inhibition of pacing in that chamber, and it will deliver a paced beat in either chamber if it does not sense an intrinsic beat. Position 4 refers to whether the rate response is turned on or off. When it is on, the atrial and ventricular rates will increase based on physiologic need. This is determined by sensors within the pacemaker.

Another commonly programmed mode is VVIR. In this mode, the pacemaker senses and paces only in the ventricle. It will inhibit pacing if an intrinsic beat is sensed. The pacemaker is programmed for the ventricle to be rate responsive, but this function is independent of the atrium in this mode. The pacemaker will allow for increased heart rate as needed during activity. This is achieved through activity and respiration sensors in the pacemaker. *Clinical Point*: This is the most common mode seen in patients with chronic atrial fibrillation.

Rate-responsive pacemakers can be programmed further to allow for mode switching. Ventricular tracking of atrial rates is desirable to allow for AV synchrony and normal response to exercise during ventricular pacing. However, if the ventricle tracks the atrium during an atrial arrhythmia, this can lead to unnecessarily elevated ventricular paced rates. Therefore, mode switching is quite useful in patients with atrial arrhythmias. The device will allow the ventricle to track the atrial rate up to a certain point, called the upper rate limit. If the device detects an atrial high rate suggestive of an atrial arrhythmia, it will then switch modes from DDDR to VVIR. The purpose of this is to avoid unnecessary ventricular tracking of elevated atrial rates. For instance, if a patient has paroxysmal atrial fibrillation, the ventricle will only track the atrium to whatever bpm the upper rate limit is set. Frequently, the upper rate limit is set at 110 bpm. At this point, the device switches to VVIR mode, and the ventricle will no longer "see" what the atrium is doing and will no longer track the atrial rate.

PACEMAKER MALFUNCTION

There are many potential problems that can result from pacemaker malfunction. Some of the more common malfunctions you should be able to pick out on an EKG are presented below.

- **Over sensing**: Pacemaker over sensing results in under pacing, as the device is sensing electrical activity that is not there and inhibiting pacing (EKG 11.8). For example, if the patient has tall T waves, these can be mistaken for R waves. The device sees this and withholds pacing. Under pacing can also occur as a result of over sensing electromagnetic interference.

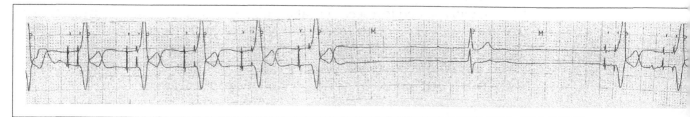

EKG 11.8

- **Under sensing or failure to sense**: This results in over pacing, as the device is not appropriately sensing intrinsic activity. It delivers unnecessary pacing spikes in the presence of intrinsic electrical activity (EKG 11.9). This can occur when there is inflammation present after a new device implant and the leads are trying to interpret intrinsic activity through scar tissue. It can also occur in lead dislodgement.

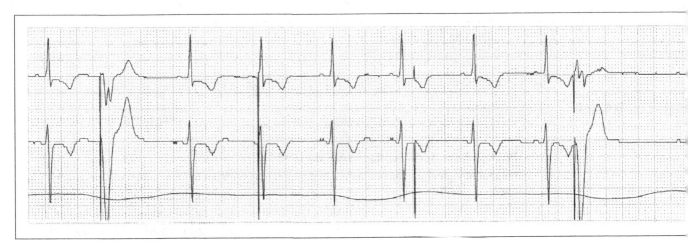

EKG 11.9

- One of the most common scenarios during which over pacing occurs as a result of under sensing is **failure to mode switch in atrial fibrillation or flutter**. Recall that a pacemaker programmed to be rate responsive will allow for ventricular tracking of an elevated atrial rate. Once it reaches the upper rate limit, it should switch modes to avoid unnecessarily high ventricular paced rates as a result of tracking. If the device fails to sense the atrial high rate, it will assume the patient is exercising or doing another activity that requires AV synchrony and an appropriate chronotropic response. This will result in abnormally high ventricular paced rates on the EKG because the device did not "see" that the atrial rate is excessively high and it fails to mode switch.

- **Failure to capture or output failure**: This occurs when there is a pacing spike but no P wave or QRS (EKG 11.10). The device is delivering a stimulus, but the energy put out is not sufficient enough to stimulate an electrical impulse. This can be seen in lead dislodgement, battery failure, an inappropriately programmed lead output, or lead fractures.

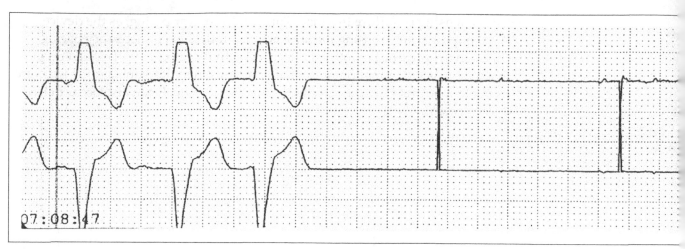

07:08:47

EKG 11.10

• **Pacemaker-mediated tachycardia (PMT)**: In normal hearts, there is a refractory period that occurs after electrical conduction, which allows for a resetting of the conduction system before another cycle takes place. In dual-chamber pacemakers, the most important refractory period is referred to as the postventricular atrial refractory period (PVARP). After a ventricular beat, the atria should be refractory, or, blinded for a period of time. During the PVARP, if a P wave occurs either from antegrade or retrograde activation, it should not be tracked by the ventricle. This would result in a paced ventricular beat. If the PVARP is not programmed correctly in a dual-chamber tracking mode, a retrograde P wave is sensed by the ventricle and a paced ventricular beat is delivered in response. The refractory period is not sufficient to allow for a blinding, or, unresponsive period that would occur with normal conduction system function. This sets up an endless loop tachycardia. The retrograde P wave is transmitted from the ventricle to the atrium via the AV node and from the atrium to the ventricle via the pacemaker as part of its tracking mode.

There are several clues on EKG or telemetry to help pick this out. First, look for a slower heart rate that immediately increases to the upper rate limit of the pacemaker, usually 110 to 120 bpm. This will be an abrupt increase, not a gradual increase that you would expect to see during sinus tachycardia. Second, look for a retrograde P wave just prior to the initiation of ventricular pacing. If a pacemaker magnet is placed over the device, this will cause asynchronous ventricular pacing at a fixed rate, which varies by device manufacturer. If there is true PMT, the loop tachycardia will be immediately terminated, and normal device function will ensue. EKG 11.11 demonstrates what PMT will look like on telemetry. EKG 11.12 is an intracardiac EKG from the same patient, taken during pacemaker interrogation. Note the initiation of the impulse in the ventricle and its retrograde transmission to the atrium. This PMT was terminated by the application of a pacemaker magnet.

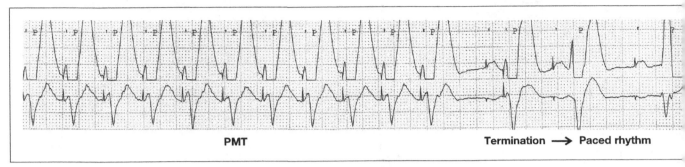

PMT   Termination ⟶ Paced rhythm

EKG 11.11

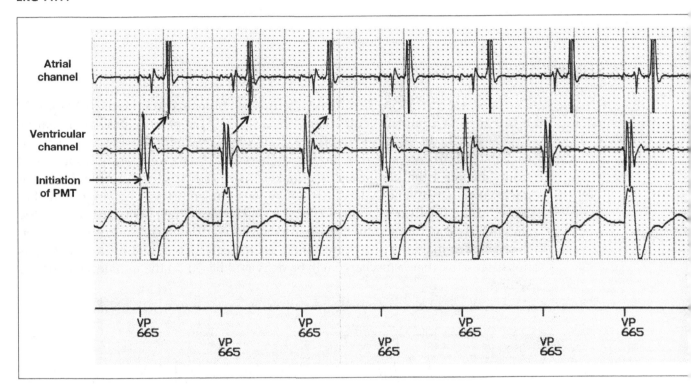

Atrial channel

Ventricular channel

Initiation of PMT ⟶

VP 665   VP 665   VP 665   VP 665   VP 665

VP 665   VP 665   VP 665

EKG 11.12

An additional, usually beneficial programmable feature is present in several device manufacturer models as part of their mode switching capability. It is frequently mistaken for pacemaker malfunction and is a common source of often unnecessary concern. This mode will allow for intermittently dropped QRS complexes while the device searches for intrinsic conduction. This mode is designed to minimize ventricular pacing and promote intrinsic conduction. When this function is available and programmed on, it essentially allows the device to briefly function as an AAI pacemaker with backup ventricular pacing while the device searches for intrinsic conduction. The dropped QRS complexes will cause a Wenckebach appearance on EKG. The key is to look for an intermittent dropped QRS complex followed by an AV-paced beat with a short AV delay. After the dropped beat, dual-chamber pacing will ensue for a period of time (EKG 11.13).

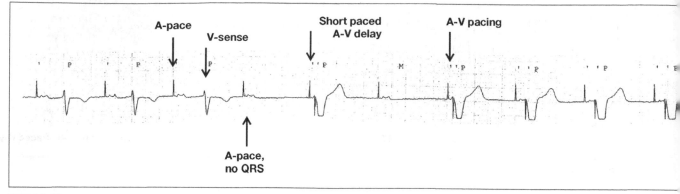

EKG 11.13

EKG FINDINGS SPECIFIC TO ICDs

The most specific pacing function of the ICD is antitachycardia pacing (ATP). ATP is designed to terminate ventricular tachycardia (VT) in place of an ICD discharge. Repeated ICD discharges may place a drain on ICD battery life and cause significant patient anxiety and discomfort. Therefore, ATP is a very useful tool. Recall from Chapter 4 that the fastest pacemaker inside the heart will be the dominant pacemaker. If a patient's VT cycle length is 160 bpm, an ICD can be programmed to sense this and deliver a round of ATP at a slightly faster rate (EKG 11.14). Note the slight increase in rate and the change in axis with ATP delivery. More often than not, this will terminate the arrhythmia and baseline conduction will resume. If ATP is not successful, then a discharge will be delivered based on the individual patient's setting.

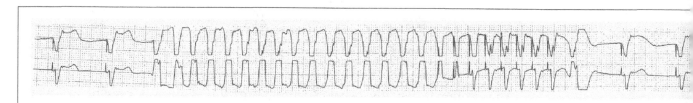

EKG 11.14

CHAPTER 11 REVIEW QUESTIONS

1. All defibrillators are also _____.

2. Right ventricular pacing results in a _____ pattern.

3. Pacemaker under sensing results in _____.

4. Pacemaker over sensing results in _____.

5. Pacemaker-mediated tachycardia can be terminated by _____.

6. ATP can terminate ventricular arrhythmias by pacing slightly _____ than the arrhythmia rate.

Drug Effects on the EKG

INTRODUCTION

The specific effect a medication will have on EKG intervals is directly related to the physiologic effect it will have on the electrical conduction system. Therefore, it is easier to understand what occurs if the medicines are thought of in groups based on their mechanism of action. Antiarrhythmic medications need to be closely monitored with regular EKGs because their effect on the conduction system can be potentially harmful.

Antiarrhythmic medications cause a change in action potentials to suppress arrhythmias. The cardiac myocyte has a negative resting charge. The myocytes become electrically excitable when there is an influx or efflux of ions from the cell. Each ion channel has a different effect on the action potential, whether it is sodium, potassium, or calcium channels. These effects are seen on the EKG by examining the intervals that reflect a specific ion channel's activity. Blocking these channels results in an interruption of reentrant mechanisms and makes it more difficult for arrhythmias to manifest.

CARDIAC ACTION POTENTIAL

The cardiac action potential is represented in Figure 12.1. During phase four, the myocyte is in a resting phase and carries a membrane potential of −90mV. In phase zero, the fast sodium channels open and sodium rushes into the cell. This causes a rapid upstroke in the action potential and the cell begins to depolarize. In phase one, potassium effluxes from the cell and the action potential increases further to 0 mV.

Phase two is the plateau phase, when potassium continues to efflux and calcium begins to influx into the cell. Phase three begins when potassium efflux exceeds the calcium influx. This causes the cell to repolarize on its way to phase four, when it again achieves a resting state and a negative membrane potential. It is these changes that are responsible for the intervals seen on an EKG. Sodium and calcium influx are the predominant players in depolarization, whereas potassium efflux is primarily responsible for repolarization. Antiarrhythmic medications alter these events at a cellular level to cause their desired effects. There is often a fine line between therapeutic and detrimental effects, and it is the job of the clinician to be able to recognize this on an EKG.

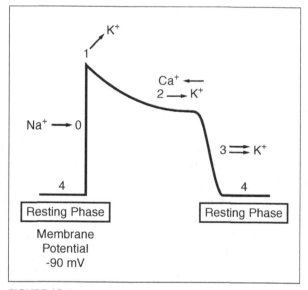

FIGURE 12.1

ANTIARRHYTHMIC CLASSES (TABLE 12.1)

- **Class I: Sodium channel blockers**

  Ia: Quinidine, procainamide, disopyramide

  - Moderate sodium channel blockade

  - Predominantly affect sodium channels; affect potassium and calcium channels to a lesser degree

  - EKG changes that may occur: QRS prolongation, QTc prolongation, and widening of P waves

  Ib: Lidocaine, phenytoin, mexiletine

  - Weak sodium channel blockade

  - EKG changes that may occur: Little to no effect on the EKG

TABLE 12.1 Antiarrhythmic Classes

Class	Action	PRi	QRS	QTc	Heart Rate
Ia	Moderate sodium blockade	_____	Increase	Increase	_____
Ic	Strong sodium blockade	Increase	Increase	Little to no effect	Decrease
II	Beta blockade	Increase	_____	_____	Decrease
III	Potassium blockade	Increase	Increase	Increase	Decrease
IV	Calcium channel blockade	Increase	_____	_____	Decrease
V	Adenosine, digoxin	Increase	_____	_____	Decrease

Ic: Flecainide, propafenone, moricizine, encainide

- Strong sodium channel blockade
- EKG changes that may occur: prolonged QRS duration or PR interval and decreased sinus rate
- Little to no effect on the QTc

- **Class II: Beta blockers**

  - Block beta adrenergic receptors
  - EKG changes that may occur: decreased sinus rate, prolonged PR interval; at higher doses, can contribute to heart block

- **Class III: Potassium channel blockers**

  - Amiodarone, sotalol, ibutilide, dofetilide, dronedarone
  - Block potassium channels and prolong repolarization
  - EKG changes that may occur: decreased sinus rate; prolonged PR interval, QRS duration, and QTc

- **Class IV: Calcium channel blockers**

  - Verapamil, diltiazem
  - Block slow calcium channels
  - EKG changes that may occur: decreased sinus rate, prolonged PR interval; at higher doses, can contribute to heart block

- **Class V: Other**

  - Adenosine, digoxin, magnesium sulfate

  - EKG changes vary by mechanism of the drug. Adenosine will slow conduction transiently within the atrioventricular (AV) node. Digoxin slows conduction through the AV node, prolongs the PR interval, and can shorten the QTc. It also causes a classic downward swooping of the ST segment that should not be confused with ST depression.

The examples below demonstrate the profound effects that antiarrhythmic medications can have on the EKG. The patient of EKG 12.1 was started on flecainide.

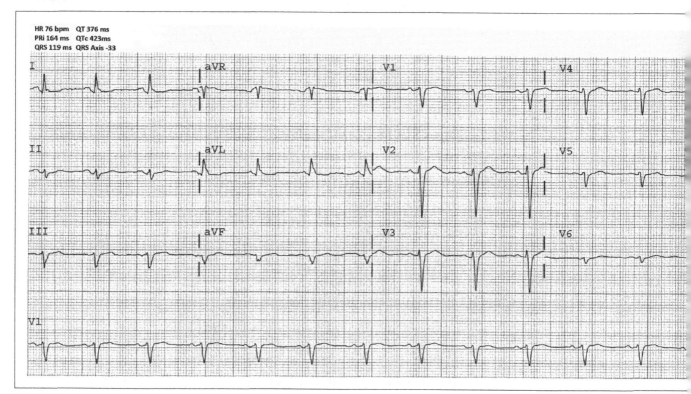

EKG 12.1

After just a few doses, there was significant widening of the QRS duration and a prolongation of the PR interval (EKG 12.2). With cessation of the drug, these intervals quickly returned to near baseline levels.

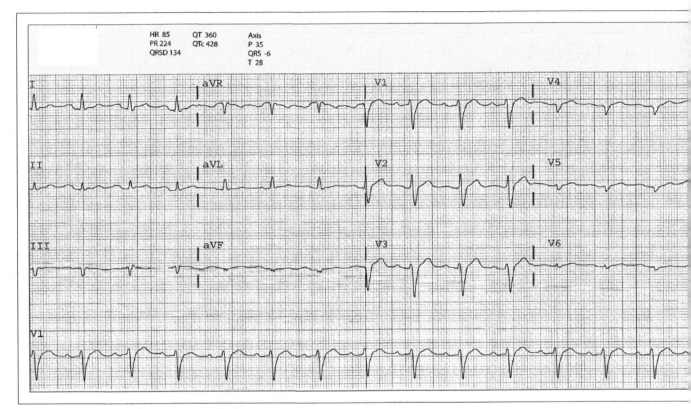

EKG 12.2

In EKG 12.3, note the extremely wide, unstable appearing QRS and the resemblance of ventricular tachycardia (VT). This pattern is sometimes referred to as a sine wave. This unfortunate patient was suffering from flecainide toxicity due to supratherapeutic doses.

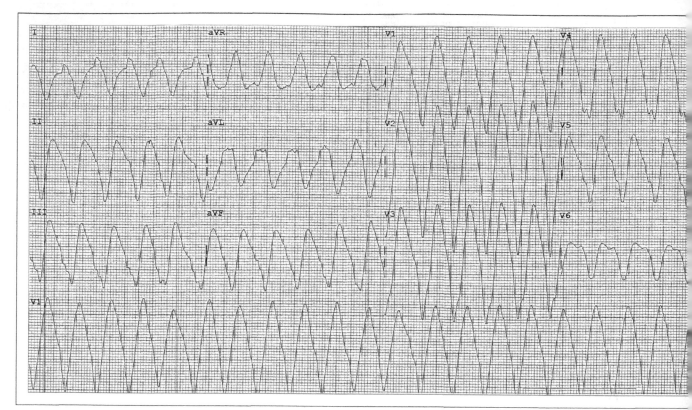

EKG 12.3

The patient of EKG 12.4 presented to the hospital with renal failure in the presence of sotalol therapy. This resulted in supratherapeutic doses of this renally excreted drug. Note the prolonged QT interval, which places the patient at risk for malignant ventricular arrhythmias.

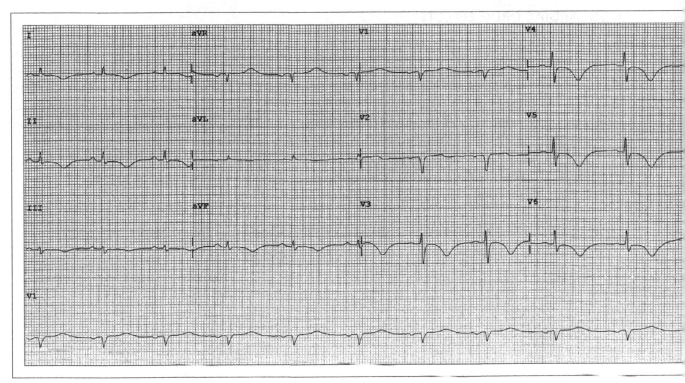

EKG 12.4

In EKG 12.5, the telemetry strip shows a prolonged QT interval in the setting of tikosyn therapy. A premature ventricular contraction falls after the apex of the T wave, and a short run of polymorphic VT occurs as a result.

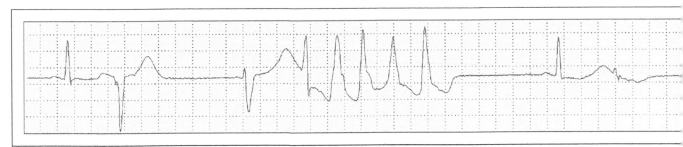

EKG 12.5

NONCARDIAC DRUG EFFECTS ON EKG

Several classes of noncardiac drugs can also affect the EKG. The most potentially dangerous effect is a prolongation of the QT interval. *Clinical Point*: Any drug that prolongs the QT interval can be associated with sudden cardiac death related to Torsades de pointes. The International Registry for Drug-Induced Arrrhythmias Arizona classification identifies many medications that can cause a prolongation of the QTc. These are further broken down into drugs that carry a conditional risk, a possible association, and a definitive association. Of commonly prescribed medicines in the general population, drugs that may prolong the QT interval include:

• Typical and atypical antipsychotics

• Antidepressants, particularly, the selective serotonin reuptake inhibitors

• Fluoroquinolone and macrolide antibiotics

• Antifungals

CHAPTER 13

Left Ventricular Hypertrophy, Electrolyte Effects, and Other Miscellaneous Findings on EKG

LEFT VENTRICULAR HYPERTROPHY

Left ventricular hypertrophy refers to an increase in size or thickness of the left ventricle (Figure 13.1). It is commonly seen in patients with conditions that place a strain on the pumping pattern of the left ventricle due to an increased pressure load. *Clinical Point*: Common conditions that lead to left ventricular hypertrophy include long-standing hypertension, valvular disorders such as aortic stenosis and aortic regurgitation, and dilated cardiomyopathy.

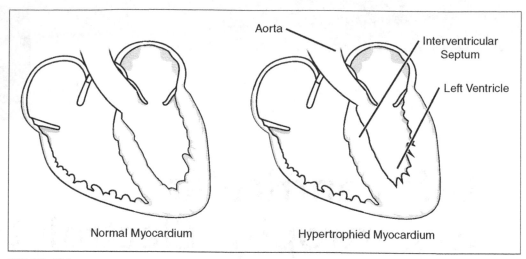

FIGURE 13.1

Evidence of left ventricular hypertrophy is particularly prominent in the precordial leads. As detailed by Surawicz and Knilans (2001), there are four main factors to look for in diagnosing left ventricular hypertrophy on EKG (EKG 13.1). These include:

- **Increased QRS voltage**

  ○ This is seen as tall QRS spikes that frequently overlap in proximal leads. The T wave will be in the opposite direction of the QRS segment in leads with increased voltage.

- **Interventricular conduction delay**

  ○ The QRS is widened but does not quite meet the criteria for a bundle branch block unless a bundle branch block is also present.

- **Repolarization abnormality** is seen as a widening of the QRS/T angle.

  ○ This occurs because of a delay in the spread of electrical impulses through the thickened myocardium.

- **Left axis deviation** may be noted as a result of the previous three criteria.

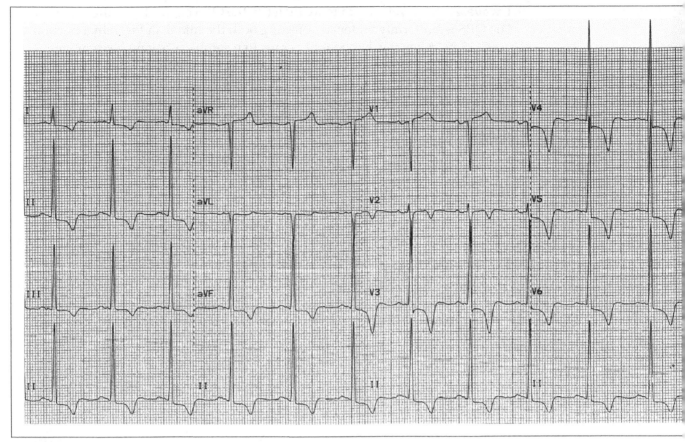

EKG 13.1

The EKG can be insensitive in diagnosing left ventricular hypertrophy. This is because the electrical activity recorded on the EKG is affected by everything that lies in between the heart and the surface electrodes. This includes adipose tissue, fluid levels such as those in pericardial and pleural effusions, and increased lung volume such as in COPD. *Clinical Point*: Left ventricular hypertrophy should not be overlooked as it is a risk factor for many cardiovascular conditions such as stroke, myocardial infarction, and heart failure. If you suspect left ventricular hypertrophy on EKG, it may lead you to order other more sensitive tests to aid in the diagnosis.

ELECTROLYTE ABNORMALITIES

An imbalance in electrolytes can lead to potentially deadly arrhythmias. It is vital to be able to quickly recognize subtle EKG changes. The main electrolytes that affect the EKG are potassium and calcium.

- **Hyperkalemia**: EKG changes begin to occur at levels more than 5.5, but are much more obvious at levels more than 6.5. The first change is a peaking of the

T wave. As the levels rise to more than 6.5, the QRS begins to be affected as well. The QRS is uniformly widened, affecting both the initial and terminal portion (EKG 13.2). When this happens, it begins to resemble a "dying heart or sine wave" pattern. There is a marked QRS prolongation with or without irregularity. Potassium levels greater than 7.0 also affect the P wave, causing a widening and flattening of the P wave with an overall decrease in amplitude. *Clinical Point*: If hyperkalemia is not corrected, it can result in heart block, ventricular fibrillation, or ventricular asystole.

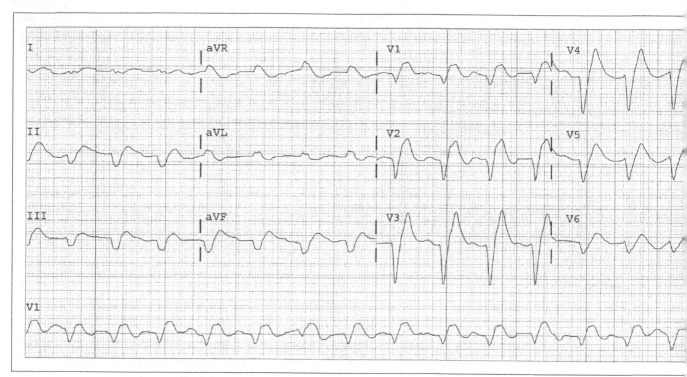

EKG 13.2

- **Hypokalemia**: EKG changes begin to occur at levels less than 3.0 and are more prominent at levels less than 2.7. Hypokalemia causes prolonged repolarization time. This leads to ST depression or T wave inversion and a prolonged QT interval (EKG 13.3). Prominent U waves may be present, sometimes becoming larger than the T wave. Other times the U wave is buried within the prolonged QT interval. These EKG changes are directly proportional to serum levels of potassium. The lower the potassium, the more prominent the changes. *Clinical Point*: If untreated, hypokalemia can lead to polymorphic ventricular tachycardia and ventricular fibrillation.

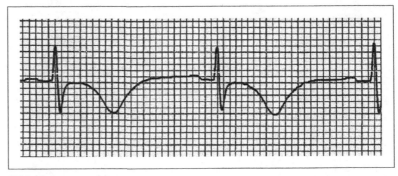

EKG 13.3

- **Hypercalcemia**: Elevated calcium levels cause a shorter ventricular repolarization time. This is seen on EKG as a subtle decrease in the QTc and a shortening of the ST segment. When serum calcium levels are significantly elevated, the T wave can appear to initiate immediately after the QRS. Despite these EKG changes, hypercalcemia has not been shown to be significantly associated with cardiac arrhythmias. *Clinical Point*: Arrhythmias can be more common in certain situations, which predispose to hypercalcemia, such as hyperparathyroid crisis.

- **Hypocalcemia**: Decreased serum calcium levels have an exact opposite effect on EKG than that described for hypercalcemia. This causes a lengthening of the ST segment and QTc. *Clinical Point*: Any time that the QTc becomes prolonged, the risk of ventricular arrhythmias is increased.

PERICARDITIS

Pericarditis is the term for inflammation of the pericardium. In the acute phase, it typically causes ST segment elevation. This can be distinguished from acute myocardial infarction by the distribution of ST changes. Because pericarditis affects the entire pericardium, ST segment elevation is usually seen in all leads. It can also cause a subtle depression below baseline in the PR interval in all leads (EKG 13.4).

In acute myocardial infarction, the ST segment elevation is localized to the offending artery's distribution site and is associated with reciprocal ST segment depression (EKG 13.5). EKG changes from pericarditis will not evolve and change with serial EKGs, in contrast to ST segment elevation in acute MI.

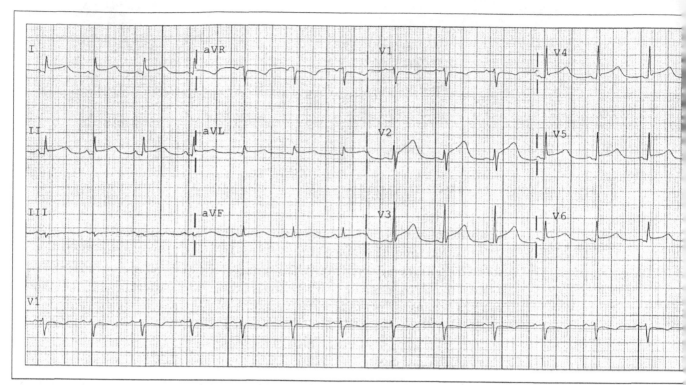

EKG 13.4

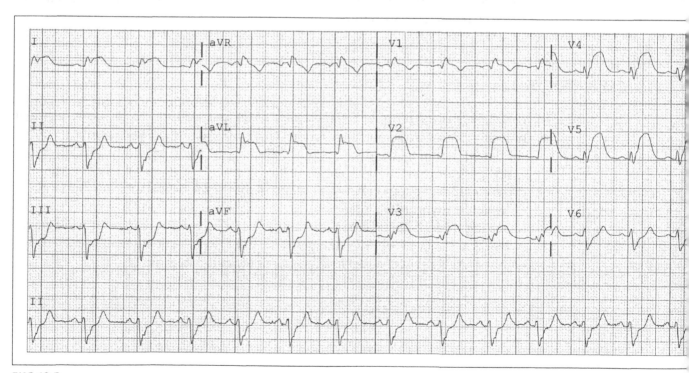

EKG 13.5

PERICARDIAL EFFUSION

Pericardial effusion occurs as a result of an abnormal collection of fluid within the pericardium. This can result in low QRS voltage in all EKG leads (EKG 13.6). If the effusion is large enough to cause a restriction of cardiac output, this is called **cardiac tamponade**, and this is a medical emergency. The classic EKG finding in the setting of cardiac tamponade is referred to as **electrical alternans**, seen as a beat-to-beat variation in the QRS axis due to a wide swinging heart within the mediastinum.

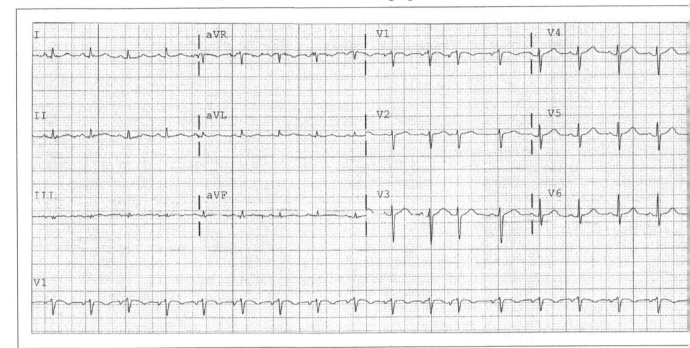

EKG 13.6

DIGOXIN

Digoxin is a medicine commonly used in the treatment of heart failure and cardiac arrhythmias and has a complex mechanism of action. The classic EKG appearance in the setting of digoxin use is the result of a change in the flow of intracardiac ions affecting both the conduction system and overall chronicity of the heart. As a result, it can shorten the repolarization time in the ventricles. This causes characteristic changes on the EKG **at normal or toxic doses**, which include

- PR interval prolongation
- ST segment depression
- A shortening of the QT interval

The most easily recognized effect is a downward swooping of the ST segment (EKG 13.7). Be careful to distinguish this finding from acute ischemia. Similar to the findings in pericarditis, ST segment depression is usually seen in all leads and will not evolve with serial EKGs.

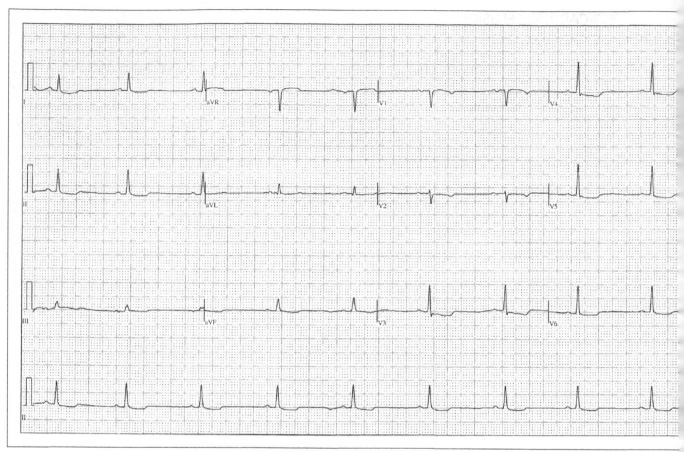

EKG 13.7

PULMONARY EMBOLISM

The EKG is not a very sensitive test for pulmonary embolism, but it can provide clues to aid in the diagnosis (EKG 13.8). There must be significant obstruction of a pulmonary artery to cause EKG changes, and even then, they can be nonspecific. These findings can also be present in other causes of cor pulmonale such as COPD, asthma, or pneumonia. The classic EKG changes can mimic inferior wall myocardial infarction. The most common findings are as follows:

- Right axis deviation with right bundle branch block or incomplete right bundle branch block pattern
- S wave in lead I, Q wave in lead III, and negative T wave in lead III due to right ventricular dilation (S1Q3T3)
- Sinus tachycardia

HYPOTHERMIA

Decreases in core body temperature have a profound effect on the conduction system. Hypothermia is associated with a lengthening of the refractory period. This

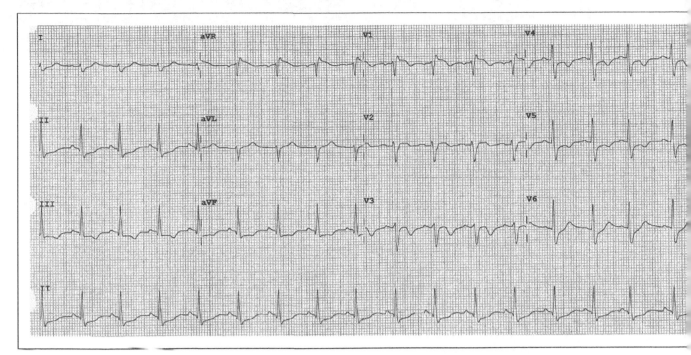

EKG 13.8

effect on EKG is seen predominantly in the ST segment. It is associated with **Osborn waves**, which are also referred to as **J waves**. This is seen as a slow upright deflection after the QRS and before the ST segment begins. J waves are best seen in the inferolateral leads and disappear with rewarming (EKG 13.9).

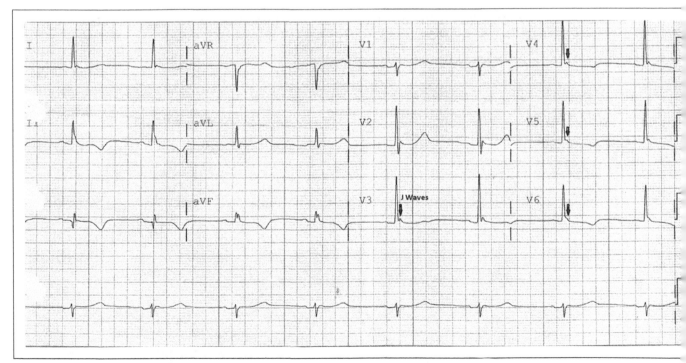

EKG 13.9

CHAPTER 13 REVIEW QUESTIONS

1. Left ventricular hypertrophy is due to a(n) _____ in left ventricular size.

2. Pulmonary embolus can cause what type of bundle branch block on EKG?

3. Is the EKG sensitive or insensitive in diagnosing left ventricular hypertrophy?

4. U waves are associated with which electrolyte abnormality?

5. Left ventricular hypertrophy is commonly associated with _____ axis deviation.

6. What effect on the QT interval does hypokalemia have?

7. The EKG hallmark of left ventricular hypertrophy is _____ QRS voltage.

8. Osborne waves are associated with _____.

14

Applying EKG Skills to Clinical Practice

After reading this book, you should feel confident in your EKG interpretation skills. As a health care provider, you must be able to appropriately and efficiently correlate subjective information with objective findings. This is especially important in EKG interpretation. In this chapter, you will be presented with a basic patient history and a corresponding EKG. Remember to follow a system so you will not leave anything out. Use the space given to document the pertinent findings. Calculate the rate in beats per minute. Evaluate if the rhythm is regular or irregular. Is the axis normal, left, or right? Look for the presence or absence of heart block. This includes sinus block; first-, second-, or third-degree atrioventricular (AV) block; bundle branch block; and QT prolongation. Look for signs of ischemia and infarction and strain patterns such as those seen in ventricular hypertrophy. After careful examination, document your final interpretation.

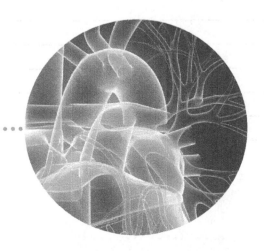

EKG 14.1

A 60-year-old female presents to the clinic for routine 6-month follow-up. She is maintained on flecainide for a history of paroxysmal atrial fibrillation. Her EKG is seen below.

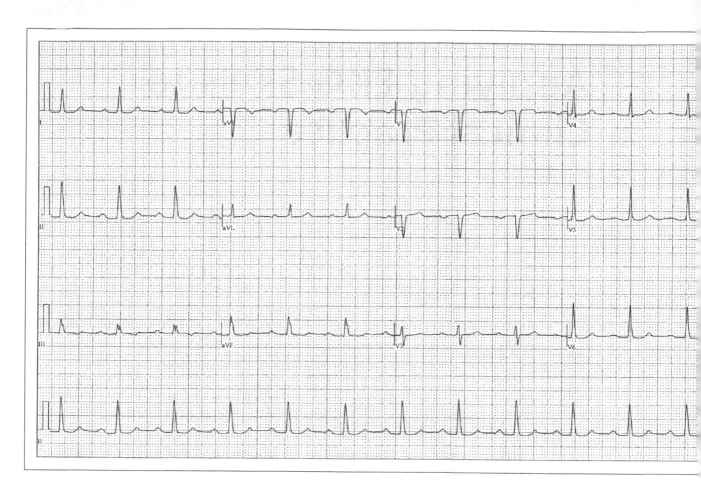

Rate: _____

Rhythm: _____

Axis: _____

Block: _____

Infarction: _____

Interpretation: _____

EKG 14.2

A 25-year-old female presents for evaluation of tachycardia and states that her heart feels like it is racing away. She has a medical history significant for generalized anxiety and feels like she may be having a panic attack. Her EKG is seen below.

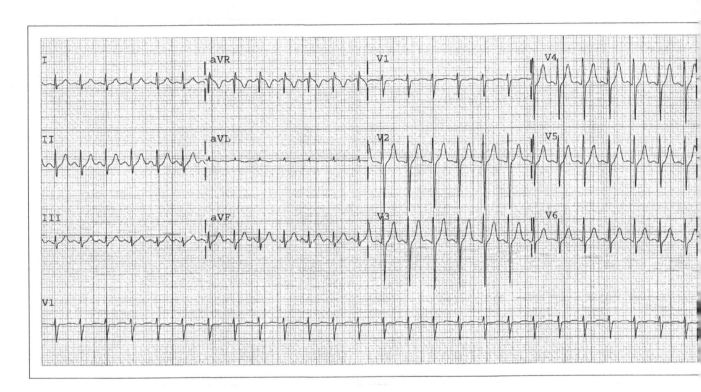

Rate: _____

Rhythm: _____

Axis: _____

Block: _____

Infarction: _____

Interpretation: _____

EKG 14.3

A 21-year-old female presents for a college sports physical and offers no complaints. An EKG is requested by her school prior to sports participation. Her EKG is seen below.

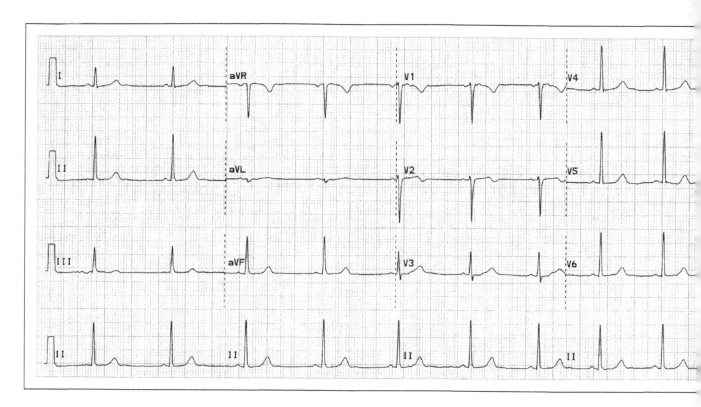

Rate: _____

Rhythm: _____

Axis: _____

Block: _____

Infarction: _____

Interpretation: _____

EKG 14.4

A 51-year-old male with a history of untreated hypertension, hyperlipidemia, and diabetes presents to the emergency department with a 30-minute history of substernal chest pressure that has been gradually getting worse. The pain began after performing strenuous yard work. His EKG is seen below.

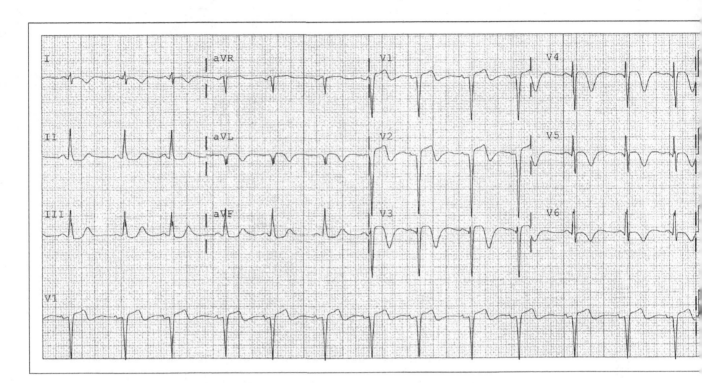

Rate: _____

Rhythm: _____

Axis: _____

Block: _____

Infarction: _____

Interpretation: _____

EKG 14.5

A 60-year-old female presents to the clinic with decreased exercise tolerance and palpitations. Her medical history is significant for mitral valve replacement 6 months ago. Her EKG is seen below.

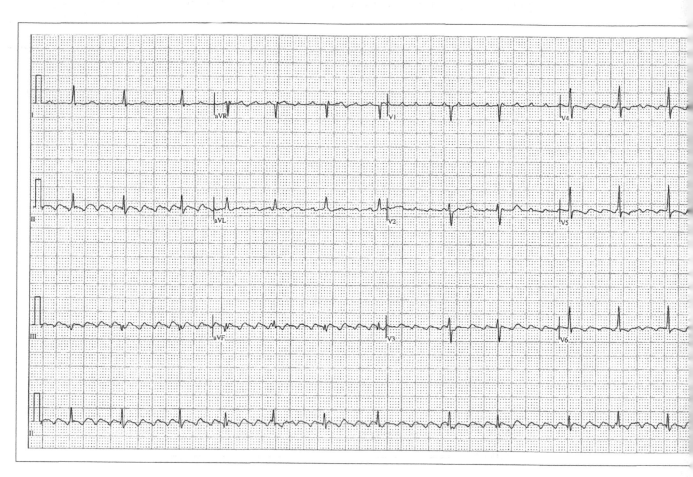

Rate: _____

Rhythm: _____

Axis: _____

Block: _____

Infarction: _____

Interpretation: _____

EKG 14.6

An 80-year-old male presents to the emergency department after experiencing a complete syncopal episode. His wife brings a copy of his medical records with her. You identify an EKG from 1 year ago documenting a left bundle branch block and first-degree AV block. His presenting EKG is shown below.

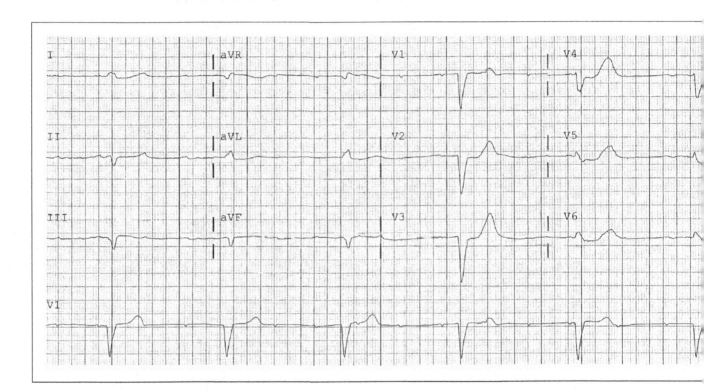

Rate: _____

Rhythm: _____

Axis: _____

Block: _____

Infarction: _____

Interpretation: _____

EKG 14.7

A 72-year-old female with a history of appropriately treated diabetes and hyperlipidemia presents to the emergency department with pain between her shoulder blades. This began 3 hours ago when she was playing outside with her grandson. The pain initially subsided with rest, but returned 1 hour ago despite rest, and is now rated an 8/10 on the pain scale. Her EKG is seen below.

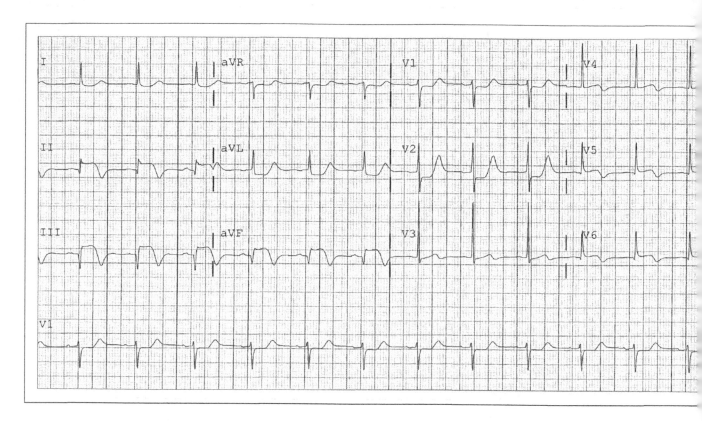

Rate: _____

Rhythm: _____

Axis: _____

Block: _____

Infarction: _____

Interpretation: _____

EKG 14.8

A 75-year-old female presents to the office for routine follow-up of obstructive sleep apnea and hypertension. Over the last several weeks, she has noted intermittent tachypalpitations. Her EKG is seen below.

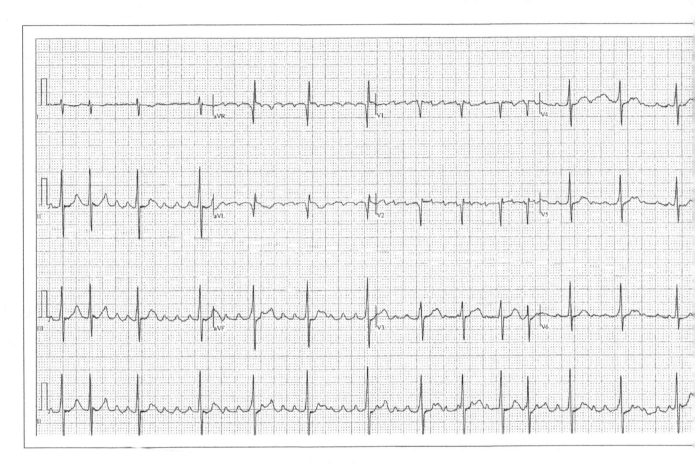

Rate: _____

Rhythm: _____

Axis: _____

Block: _____

Infarction: _____

Interpretation: _____

EKG 14.9

A 69-year-old male with a history of a newly diagnosed dilated cardiomyopathy presents for follow-up to the heart failure clinic and offers no complaints. Routine EKG is ordered to follow-up on medication changes made at last visit. His EKG is seen below.

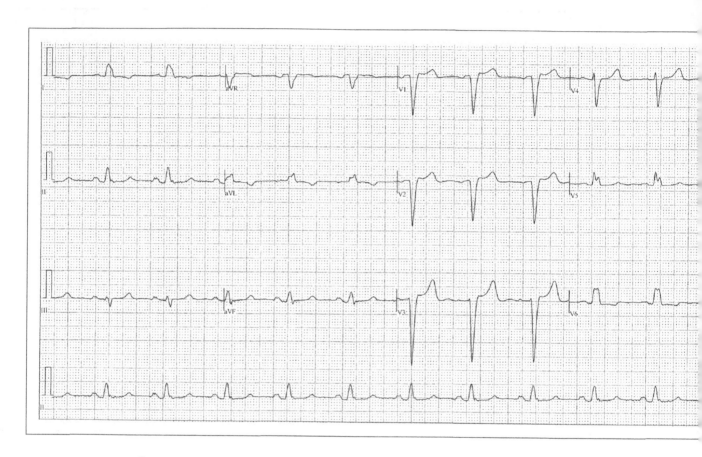

Rate: _____

Rhythm: _____

Axis: _____

Block: _____

Infarction: _____

Interpretation: _____

EKG 14.10

A 55-year-old male presents to the clinic for routine follow-up of coronary artery disease. Interpret his EKG and include the specific site of his previous myocardial infarction.

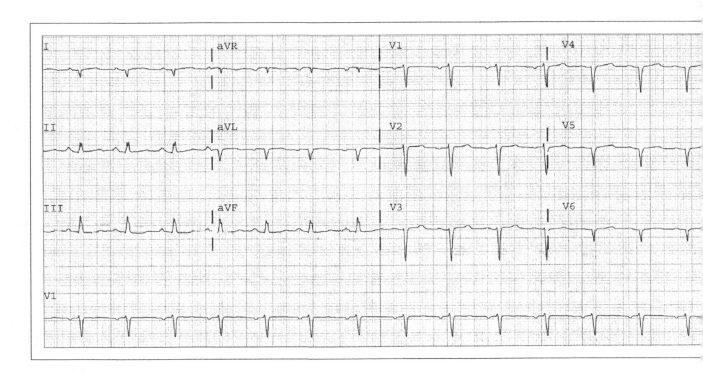

Rate: _____

Rhythm: _____

Axis: _____

Block: _____

Infarction: _____

Interpretation: _____

EKG 14.11

A 70-year-old male presents to the emergency department with tachypalpitations and diaphoresis. He is unable to give any other additional history. His EKG is seen below.

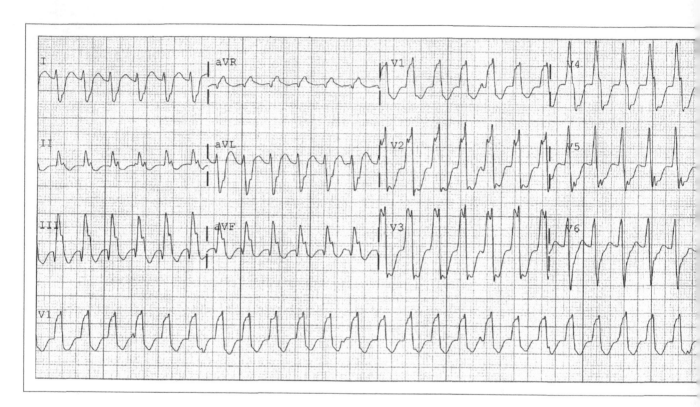

Rate: _____

Rhythm: _____

Axis: _____

Block: _____

Infarction: _____

Interpretation: _____

EKG 14.12

An 85-year-old female is seen in the outpatient clinic with intermittent lightheadedness. This occurs only when she is seated and she has come close to passing out several times in the last few days. Her EKG is seen below.

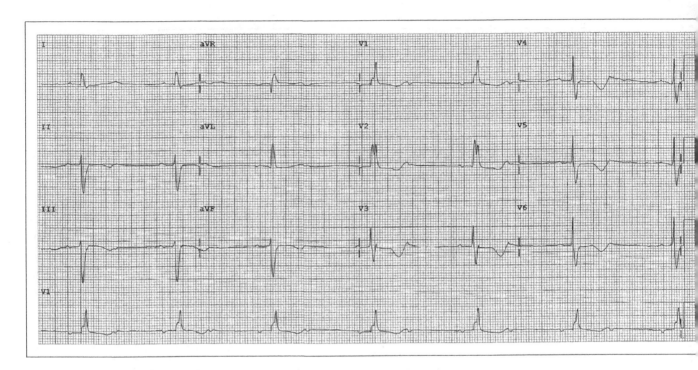

Rate: _____

Rhythm: _____

Axis: _____

Block: _____

Infarction: _____

Interpretation: _____

EKG 14.13

A 66-year-old female is seen in the outpatient clinic with increased fatigue and shortness of breath. She is usually very active and has been unable to participate in her normal aerobics class due to the dyspnea. Her EKG is seen below.

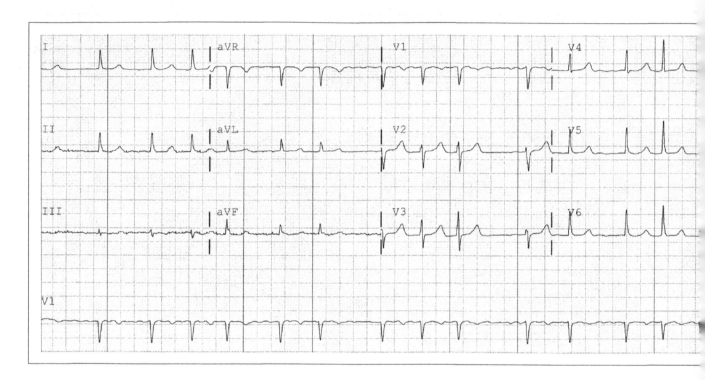

Rate: _____

Rhythm: _____

Axis: _____

Block: _____

Infarction: _____

Interpretation: _____

EKG 14.14

A 75-year-old male presents to the emergency department with progressively worsening fatigue and weakness. He has a history of hypertension, and his primary care provider recently doubled his beta blocker. His EKG is seen below.

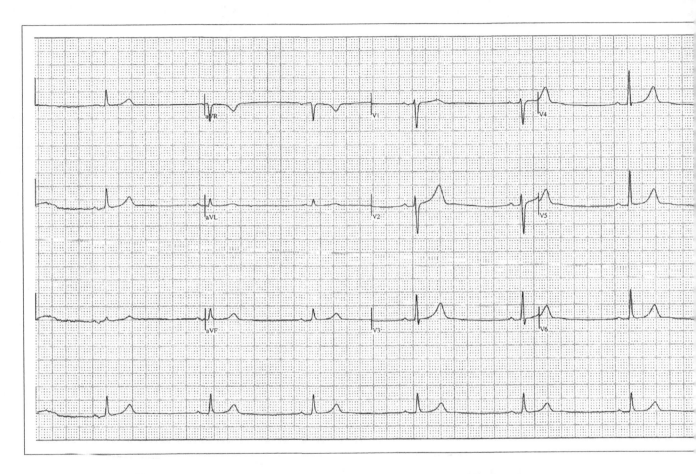

Rate: _____

Rhythm: _____

Axis: _____

Block: _____

Infarction: _____

Interpretation: _____

EKG 14.15

A 55-year-old male with a family history of coronary artery disease presents for his annual follow-up. He has no complaints. An EKG is done as a part of his annual physical and is seen below.

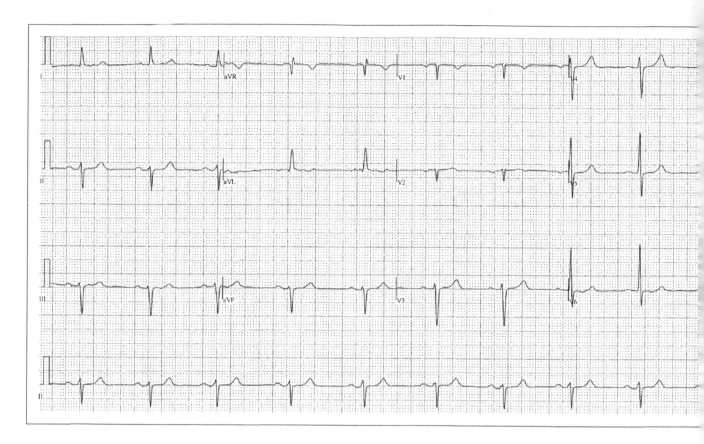

Rate: _____

Rhythm: _____

Axis: _____

Block: _____

Infarction: _____

Interpretation: _____

EKG 14.16

A 52-year-old male presents to the office with a chief complaint of palpitations. He feels that his heart is skipping "almost constantly." His symptoms worsen at night when he is relaxed and seem to improve somewhat when he is active. His EKG is seen below.

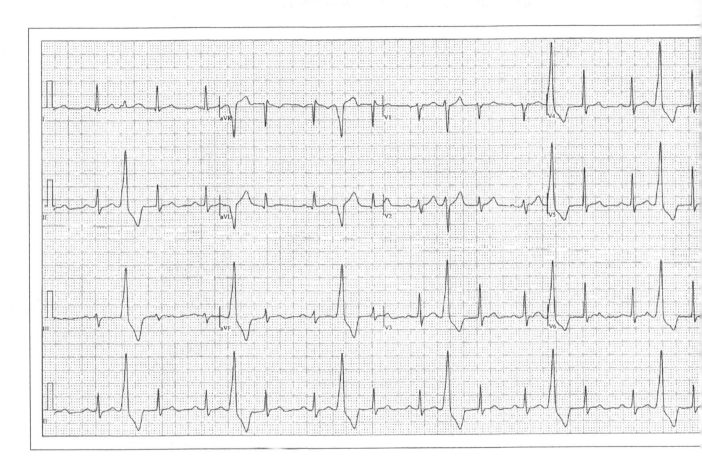

Rate: _____

Rhythm: _____

Axis: _____

Block: _____

Infarction: _____

Interpretation: _____

EKG 14.17

A 62-year-old obese male smoker with no regular medical care is brought to the emergency department by his family with active chest pain and diaphoresis. On further questioning, he has been having predictable angina symptoms for the last 5 days. The pain became so severe the morning of his presentation that he agreed to come to the hospital. His EKG is seen below.

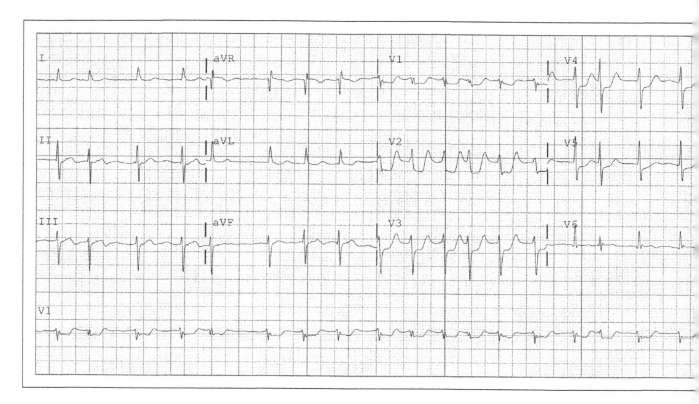

Rate: _____

Rhythm: _____

Axis: _____

Block: _____

Infarction: _____

Interpretation: _____

EKG 14.18

A 50-year-old male with paroxysmal atrial fibrillation treated with sotalol presents to the outpatient clinic after experiencing several episodes of chest discomfort and near syncope. He was recently prescribed levofloxacin for pneumonia, and his symptoms began 2 days after starting this new medication. His EKG is seen below.

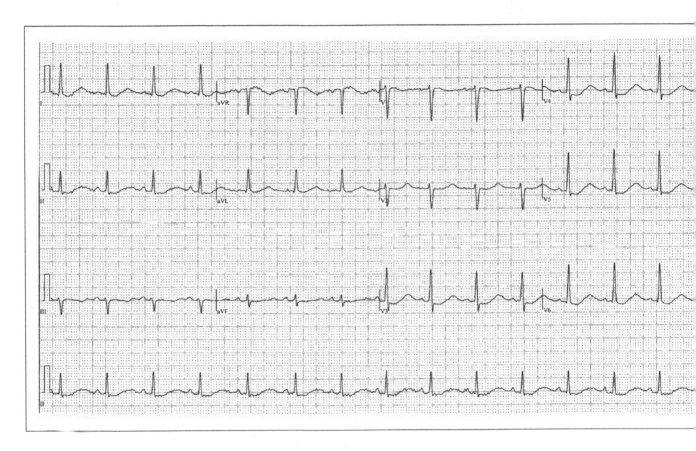

Rate: _____

Rhythm: _____

Axis: _____

Block: _____

Infarction: _____

Interpretation: _____

Resources

Bonow, R. O., Mann, D. L., Zipes, D. P., & Libby, P. (2012). *Braunwald's heart disease: A textbook of cardiovascular medicine* (9th ed.). Philadelphia, PA: Saunders.

Braunwald, E. (Ed.). (2001). *Harrison's principles of internal medicine* (15th ed.). New York, NY: McGraw-Hill.

Chow, A. E., & Buxton, A. (2006). *Implantable cardiac pacemakers and defibrillators all you wanted to know*. Malden, MA: Blackwell Publishing.

Crawford, M. (2009). *Current diagnosis and treatment cardiology* (3rd ed.). New York, NY: McGraw-Hill Companies.

Crawford, P. (Ed.). (2004). *The Washington manual cardiology subspecialty consult*. Philadelphia, PA: Lippincott Williams and Wilkins.

Dubin, D. (1999). *Rapid interpretation of EKG's* (5th ed.). Tampa, FL: Cover.

Epstein, A. E., DiMarco, J. P., Ellenbogen, K. A., Estes, N. A., III, Freedman, R. A., Gettes, L. S., ... Yancy, C. W. (2008). ACC/AHA/HRS 2008 guidelines for device-based therapy of cardiac rhythm abnormalities: A report of the American College of Cardiology/American Heart Association Task Force. *Journal of American College of Cardiology*, 51(21), e1–e62.

Gage, B. F., Waterman, A. D., Shannon, W., Boechler, M., Rich, M. W., & Radford, M. J. (2001). Validation of clinical classification schemes for predicting stroke. Results from the national registry of atrial fibrillation. *Journal of the American Medical Association*, 285(22), 2864–2870.

Goldberger, A. (1999). *Clinical electrocardiography a simplified approach* (6th ed.). St. Louis, MO: Mosby.

Sgarbossa, E. B., Pinski, S. L., Gates, K. B., & Wagner, G. S. (1996). Early electrocardiographic diagnosis of acute myocardial infarction in the presence of ventricular paced rhythm. GUSTO-I investigators. *American Journal of Cardiology*, 77(5), 423–424.

Shantsila, E., Watson, T., & Lip, G. Y. (2007). Drug induced QT interval prolongation and proarrhythmic risk in the treatment of atrial arrhythmias. *Europace*, 9(4), 37–44.

Surawicz, B., & Knilans, T. (2001). *Chou's electrocardiography in clinical practice* (5th ed). Philadelphia, PA: Saunders.

Jolly, K., Gammage, M.D., Cheng, K.K., Bradburn, P., Banting, M.V., Langman, M.J. (2009). Sudden death in patients receiving drugs tending to prolong the QT interval. *Br J Clin Pharmacol*, 68(5), 743–751.

Wagner, G. (2007). *Marriot's practical electrocardiography* (11th ed.). Philadelphia, PA: Lippincott Williams and Wilkins.

Wellens, H. J., Bar, F. W., & Lie, J. I. (1978). The value of the electrocardiogram in the differential diagnosis of a tachycardia with a widened QRS complex. *American Journal of Medicine, 64*(1), 27–33.

Answer Key

CHAPTER 1
1. 60 and 100 bpm
2. Positive
3. Negative
4. Negative
5. Anterior and posterior
6. AV node
7. Purkinje fibers

CHAPTER 2
1. 120–200 milliseconds
2. 80–120 milliseconds
3. Less than 440–460 milliseconds
4. Ventricular arrhythmias
5. QT interval
6. J point
7. Bradycardia
8. Apex of the T wave

CHAPTER 3
1. I, II, and III
2. aVR, aVL, and aVF
3. II and III
4. I and III
5. I and II
6. Positive
7. Negative
8. V4

CHAPTER 4
1. 60 and 100 bpm
2. 40 and 60 bpm
3. 20 and 40 bpm
4. 40 bpm, ventricles
5. 50 bpm, sinus node

CHAPTER 5
1. Regular
2. Irregularly irregular
3. Irregular, P waves
4. Atrial bigeminy
5. Decrease

CHAPTER 6
1. Left axis deviation: −60 degrees
   Right axis deviation: +90 degrees
   Normal axis: +30 degrees

CHAPTER 7
1. 100 milliseconds
2. Mobitz I second degree
3.A. Left bundle branch block
3.B. Left anterior fascicular block
3.C. Right bundle branch block
4. Complete
5. Left
6. Right
7. Mobitz II

CHAPTER 8
1. Ischemia
2. Q waves
3. Left bundle branch block
4. V1–V4 and II, III, aVF
5. II, III, aVF and I, aVL
6. I, aVL, V5–V6 and II, III, aVF
7. ST segment elevation
8.A. Right coronary artery
8.B. Left circumflex

CHAPTER 9
1. Slow and a fast pathway
2. P waves, irregular
3. Negative, positive
4. Pre-excitation
5. AV node
6. Accessory pathway
7. Stroke

CHAPTER 10
1. A-V dissociation
2. Monomorphic
3. Torsades de pointes
4. Ventricular fibrillation
5. Direct current cardioversion
6. Multifocal
7. Ventricular tachycardia

CHAPTER 11
1. Pacemakers
2. Left bundle branch block
3. Over pacing
4. Under pacing
5. Placing a pacemaker magnet over the device
6. Faster

CHAPTER 13
1. Increase
2. Right bundle branch block
3. Insensitive
4. Hypokalemia
5. Left
6. Prolongation of the QT interval
7. Increased
8. Hypothermia

CHAPTER 14
EKG 14.1
Rate: 75 bpm
Rhythm: Regular, sinus
Axis: Normal
Block: First-degree AVB with PRi approximately 280 milliseconds
Infarction: None
Interpretation: Normal sinus rhythm with first-degree AV block

EKG 14.2
Rate: 150 bpm
Rhythm: Regular, sinus
Axis: Normal
Block: None
Infarction: None
Interpretation: Sinus tachycardia

EKG 14.3
Rate: 55 bpm
Rhythm: Regular, sinus
Axis: Normal
Block: None

EKG 14.3 (cont.)

Infarction: None

Interpretation: Mild sinus bradycardia within normal limits for a trained athlete

EKG 14.4

Rate: 80 bpm

Rhythm: Regular, sinus

Axis: Borderline right axis deviation. Lead I is isoelectric placing the axis at approximately +90 degrees

Block: Slight prolongation of the QTc. Note that the QT interval is slightly more than half the R-R interval in most leads.

Infarction: Anteroseptal ST elevation and T wave inversion involving the anterior and lateral leads

Interpretation: Acute myocardial ischemia involving the anterolateral leads. This is causing a slight prolongation of the QTc and delayed R wave transition in the precordial leads.

EKG 14.5

Rate: Approximately 70 bpm

Rhythm: Irregularly irregular involving repetitive cycles. This is due to variable block in the setting of atrial flutter. The flutter waves are negative in leads II, III, and aVF and positive in lead V1.

Axis: Normal axis. aVF is predominantly positive, although the QRS is partially obscured by the flutter waves. Lead I is positive.

Block: None, although the flutter waves are blocking in a variable 3:1 to 4:1 pattern.

Infarction: None evident

Interpretation: Typical atrial flutter with a controlled, variable ventricular response

EKG 14.6

Rate: 30 bpm

Rhythm: Regular, sinus

Axis: Left axis. aVR is most isoelectric placing the axis at approximately −60

Block: Complete AV block

Infarction: Cannot reliably evaluate for ischemia in the setting of a ventricular escape rhythm.

Interpretation: Complete AV block with a ventricular junctional escape at a rate of 30 bpm

EKG 14.7

Rate: 75 bpm

Rhythm: Regular, sinus

Axis: Left axis. Lead II is the most isoelectric placing the axis at approximately −30 degrees

Block: None

Infarction: 3–4 mm ST segment elevation in the inferior leads with reciprocal ST depression in the lateral leads. There is 1–2 mm ST depression in the anteroseptal leads as well.

Interpretation: Acute inferior wall myocardial infarction with probable early posterior involvement

EKG 14.8

Rate: Approximately 70 bpm

Rhythm: Irregularly irregular consistent with atrial flutter with variable block. P waves are positive in leads II, III, aVF, and V1.

Axis: Right axis. Lead I is predominantly negative and lead aVF is predominantly positive. Leads II and aVR are isoelectric, placing the axis between +120 and +150 degrees.

Block: None, although the atrial flutter is occurring with a variable 3:1 to 4:1 block.

Infarction: None

Interpretation: Atypical atrial flutter with variable block and a controlled ventricular response of 80 bpm

EKG 14.9

Rate: 70 bpm

Rhythm: Regular, sinus

EKG 14.9 (cont.)

Axis: Normal

Block: Left bundle branch block pattern is evident on examination of leads V1 and V6. There is also a borderline first-degree AV block with a PRi of 200 milliseconds

Infarction: None evident

Interpretation: Normal sinus rhythm with left bundle branch block and borderline first-degree AV block

EKG 14.10

Rate: 80 bpm

Rhythm: Regular, sinus

Axis: Right axis. Lead I is negative and lead aVF is positive. Lead aVR has both positive and negative forces, placing the axis at approximately +120 degrees

Block: No evidence of heart block. The negative forces in leads I and aVL are the result of Q waves from an old lateral wall MI, not from a true posterior fascicular block, which would cause an rS pattern in these leads.

Infarction: Q waves are predominantly seen in the lateral leads with anterior involvement causing poor R wave progression in the precordial leads.

Interpretation: Old anterolateral wall MI causing poor R wave progression across the precordial leads

EKG 14.11

Rate: 150 bpm

Rhythm: Regular with evidence of A-V dissociation

Axis: Right axis. Lead I is negative and lead aVF is positive. Lead aVR is most isoelectric placing the axis at approximately +120 degrees.

Block: Right bundle branch block pattern. Evidence of A-V dissociation is noted with visible P waves in several leads.

Infarction: Unable to evaluate given the rapid rate and wide QRS

Interpretation: Rapid monomorphic ventricular tachycardia with a right bundle branch block pattern

EKG 14.12

Rate: 35 bpm

Rhythm: Regular. P waves noted in 2:1 pattern with QRS

Axis: Left axis. Lead aVR is the most isoelectric placing the axis at approximately −60 degrees

Block: Right bundle branch block, left anterior fascicular block with 2:1 AV block

Infarction: T waves are inverted in several leads, likely the result of the ventricular conduction delay.

Interpretation: 2:1 AV block with right bundle branch block and left anterior fascicular block

EKG 14.13

Rate: 75 bpm

Rhythm: Irregularly irregular without identifiable P waves

Axis: Normal

Block: None

Infarction: None

Interpretation: Atrial fibrillation with a variable but controlled ventricular response

EKG 14.14

Rate: 30 bpm

Rhythm: Regular with sinus activity and AV association

Axis: Normal

Block: Borderline first degree AV block

Infarction: None

Interpretation: Sinus bradycardia with slow ventricular response

EKG 14.15

Rate: 60 bpm

Rhythm: Regular, sinus

Axis: Left axis. Lead aVR is most isoelectric placing the axis at approximately −60 degrees

EKG 14.15 (*cont.*)

Block: Left anterior fascicular block. Note the rS pattern in leads II, III, and aVF; tall R waves in leads I and aVL; and an axis more negative than −30 to −45 degrees.

Infarction: None.

Interpretation: Sinus rhythm with left anterior fascicular block

EKG 14.16

Rate: Intrinsic rate 80 bpm, not accounting for ectopy

Rhythm: Regularly irregular

Axis: Normal. Lead III is most isoelectric placing the axis at approximately +30 degrees

Block: None

Infarction: None

Interpretation: Normal sinus rhythm with unifocal ventricular trigeminy

EKG 14.17

Rate: Approximately 100 bpm

Rhythm: Irregularly irregular consistent with atrial fibrillation

Axis: Left axis. Lead II is the most isoelectric placing the axis at approximately −30 degrees

Block: Left anterior fascicular block

Infarction: ST depression and positive mirror sign in V1 to V3 consistent with posterior wall ischemia

Interpretation: Atrial fibrillation with slightly accelerated ventricular response, left anterior fascicular block, and acute posterior wall ischemia

EKG 14.18

Rate: 80 bpm

Rhythm: Normal sinus

Axis: Normal. Lead aVF is most isoelectric placing the axis at approximately 0 degrees

Block: The QT interval is prolonged >500 milliseconds. Note that the QT interval is greater than half the R-R interval.

Infarction: None

Interpretation: Normal sinus rhythm with a prolonged QT interval, likely secondary to concomitant sotalol and levofloxacin use

Index